# MY
# MAD
# DAD

ROBYN HOLLINGWORTH

# MY MAD DAD

TRAPEZE

First published in Great Britain in 2017 by Trapeze,
an imprint of The Orion Publishing Group Ltd
Carmelite House, 50 Victoria Embankment,
London EC4Y 0DZ

An Hachette UK company

1 3 5 7 9 10 8 6 4 2

A CIP catalogue record for this book is
available from the British Library.

ISBN (Hardback): 978 1 409 18001 2
ISBN (eBook): 978 1 409 18003 6

Typeset by Born Group

Printed and bound by CPI Group (UK) Ltd, Croydon, CR0 4YY

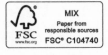

www.orionbooks.co.uk

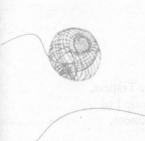

For My Mad Dad

# Introduction

## Before

I was lucky enough to be a little girl who idolised her daddy. There was much to idolise. My dad, David Coles, was a charmingly intelligent, self-made man who made people laugh and did great things. He was a civil engineer and he built power stations all over the world. He gave people power, isn't that great? He brought light into people's lives, and light into mine, in a different way.

He himself was quite a powerful man, not in an American president kind of way, just short and stocky, the sort that looked like he could handle himself if the situation might call for it. Welsh men are often short, or so my mother would tell us, and by age 14 I was as tall as he was – a grand 5 foot 8 and proud of it. Though where I was a long and lanky streak of piss (Dad's words), he was thickset and muscular, with a beard and moustache combo that had seen him through the decades when that was considered a good look, as well as those years that did not celebrate it with quite so much fervour. As he turned from young man to old, the only thing that changed about him was the colour of his facial hair, gently fading from mouse-brown to steel to placid pale grey. I remember being round at a friend's house and having fish fingers for our tea, and when she got the card container out of the freezer she pointed at the smiling chap on the logo and doubled over with euphoric childish laughter. 'Ha – look, it's your dad!' she exclaimed with glee. Captain bloody Birds Eye.

Dad's work spread far and wide, his fair and well-skilled hands touching projects all over the world, and, as a result, our family upbringing, especially in the early years, was peripatetic. We moved from country to country, from strange place to strange place, from desert to jungle, and then to Wales (Pontypool, to be precise), where my brother Gareth and I went to school. Wales, where a large part of my heart still lies, irrelevant of my current postal address. It seemed like an odd choice considering my brother had been born in Kenya and me in Dubai, but Dad had got some consulting work with a local company and they had both wanted us to be schooled in the UK. Dad was Welsh, so it seemed as good a choice as any as we approached school age. They hadn't bought into the idea of international schools for us, and I'm glad about that. They wanted us to have proper roots, and that's what they gave us. We always knew he was proud of the green green grass of home, and we all feel a strong connection with the land of song and the home of dragons.

My mum, Marjorie, as always, played the great supporting actress role. A Scot by birth and heritage, she had her own attachment to hills and valleys; well, lochs and glens, I guess, the countryside of her childhood bathed in heather and views of Aran. I suppose their upbringings kind of mirrored each other, at different ends of the country, where the working classes were just the same – strongly moralled and mute in the face of parental authority, but with the gusto and courage that puts fire in the belly and a backbone in the workforce. A wonderful and fiercely intelligent woman in her own right, Mum left bonny Scotland after school and graduated from a London university with a degree in botany. Mum and Dad met in Chelsea in the late 1960s, a fact that almost made me think they might once have been cool. They were married in a church just behind Harrods. At my first job as a buyer's assistant with Armani (you can only imagine how that news went down in Pontypool!), I would look out from the kitchen window while making tea for my boss and would always see a Scottish flag protruding from the vast, urban rooftop vista. One evening on a phone call to Mum, I told her so, and she replied, matter-of-factly, that it would be the church they married in, just behind my Knightsbridge office. After that, I would take my packed lunch and sit in the church on a Friday, thinking of them.

In the early years of their marriage, she would often take a call from our father when he would say where he had been posted to or stationed, initially as part of the Merchant Navy – his route out of the Rhondda Valley and his path to global discovery. Then she would proceed to 'pack the things and bring the children'. She put her career aside to join him on his life adventure – and what adventures we had.

Once we had settled in my father's native Wales, he continued to travel, consulting for international organisations and developing his own companies and initiatives. He was ever the entrepreneur. His desire to learn, to know, to travel and to experience was something we all lived with and shared. We would go with him, as far as school schedules allowed. This proved to be something of a novelty at a state school in a relatively poor area. My tales of trains across China for days on end, where the only loo was a rickety hole over the rails, speeding fast just inches away from my terrified little clenching bottom, and roaring lions in Africa hungrily prowling the grounds of my dad's Ugandan home always amused my schoolmates, but many of them never truly believed me. Yet when people met Dad they knew; they knew he was the real deal. He knew stuff that so many people didn't; he had been there, seen it, done it, lived it, breathed it – not in an arrogant way, he just . . . had.

You know when you grow up you think everyone is pretty much the same, that you've got what everyone else has, that beautiful and youthful innocence that is blind to difference? Well, that was tested the first time I had a group of friends come round to our house when we settled in Wales. We had a house on a nice street overlooking some fields, big enough to accommodate all our weird and wonderful artefacts from our worldly travels. Mum opened the door and in we tumbled, all messy hair and dirty jumpers, ready for racing around in the back garden before sandwiches and milk. And I watched as their childish eyes widened and their mouths fell open, stubby teeth protruding and chubby brows furrowing. 'Why do you have weapons?' one asked, pointing at the tribal spears hanging by the dining table. 'Are these things dead or alive?' asked another, breath steaming up the glass cases of Papua New Guinean butterflies and beetles. 'Can I play that guitar thing?' another one asked, with their clammy stubby fingers reaching for a rare sitar above a fireplace. Fortunately, I was a quick thinker, and I spun it so that it got around I lived in a 'fun-house', not that our family was a freak show.

The next year, I had a birthday party in the house, and while my dad sat alone in the child-free quiet of the shed drinking cans of Brains Bitter, my mum created the most magnificent treasure hunt around the house, where we had to count animal statues, list colours of exotic birds on paintings, and name countries from the globes in our bedrooms. They are the reason why my brother and I have such an encyclopaedic knowledge of the bizarre and unrelatable: capital cities of forgotten countries, Latin names for rare flowers, collective nouns for extinct species.

The older I get, the more people say I look like my mum. I guess this happens to many people and it's better than saying I look like my dad. No young woman wants that, especially when your dad looks like Captain Birds Eye. Mum's tall, slightly taller than Dad on a good day, especially with heels (her, not him) and an all-round good sort; clever, kind, charming but not afraid to speak her mind. A classic mum, homely and resourceful, kind and nurturing. I would say, though, that personality-wise, I am Dad and my brother is Mum.

Having a brother nearly five years older served me well. He was popular at school and around town, and had lots of friends. Everyone liked Gareth, and they still do. From quite early on, Dad referred to him as 'big G', and so he was usually that, just G. With an old head on young shoulders, he's responsible and caring, forward-thinking and wise. He got a paper round as soon as he was able, always wanting to work, to earn, to self-sustain. I would hear him getting ready, putting on his tracksuit and trainers with Madonna's 'Dear Jessie' a distant murmur in the background. I guess it was a radio hit at the time but I later recall him having *Immaculate Collection* on tape (he also has a penchant for Simply Red, which is, frankly, unforgivable). As the song would end he'd gently push open the door to my room, dim lamp glow from the hallway seeping onto my pillow, and ask me if I wanted to go with him. I always would. He'd wheel me to the shops on the crossbar of his bike in the pale, quiet light of morning, and would buy me a can of 7Up, because I liked the Fido Dido character, and a Marathon (before they became Snickers – a disastrous move, if you ask me). He would also give me half of his wages, despite the fact that I never delivered a single paper. That kind of sums him up: he is my protector, my strength and shield, the most perfect embodiment of a big brother. All that is good about that term was made for him.

In time, both G and I left home for university. I couldn't wait to leave home; I never wanted to stay in Pontypool indefinitely. I loved the thought of learning more, of meeting new people and seeing new things. I loved being around people from different backgrounds and hearing their stories. Being in halls at Royal Holloway University in Egham, so close to London, was exactly what I wanted, taking the train into Waterloo at weekends and just wandering round town, even with no money, was fun. Mum and Dad encouraged us to go to uni and it felt like they couldn't wait to be alone again, though I now know that after they dropped me at the haughtily beautiful Royal Holloway University Mum stopped the car at the top of the campus and cried helplessly onto Dad's shoulder. Later, Mum told me she suffered with empty nest syndrome. While gardening her way through the lonely late autumn of my first term away, she befriended a little robin who got bolder each day until he eventually sat on her basket, then trowel, then hand and tweeted kindly. She said that he made her feel like I was still there, saying hello.

I guess my parents instilled in both my brother and me the desire to seek out more than what you are raised with, encouraged us to learn about the unknown. It never occurred to us to stay put. I suppose when you travel a lot as a youngster it isn't scary to get out there; finding ways to communicate with people in a different language was an amusing and entertaining skill (we are all also highly successful at charades), and eating new foods, seeing new things and smelling new smells was so normal that the thought of never seeing 'new' probably scared and bored us in equal measure. Many of our friends who didn't move away eagerly at 18 had more roots, I guess, living on the same street as aunties and uncles, grandparents and godparents – that must make moving on more difficult, more political.

And so, from the age of 18, I lived in London, first at uni and then working as a fashion buyer after I graduated with a degree in Politics and Economics. Meanwhile, my brother chose a career as a hotelier, working in some wonderful hotels across the UK. Mum and Dad stayed in Wales but moved to a slightly smaller house further up the valley. Mum worked for a local charity, the Women's Royal Voluntary Service (WRVS), while Dad retired in his late 50s, spending his time running and keeping fit, watching club rugby, tracking his speed at *The Times* crossword and reading *Private Eye*, his head bent over our dining table, which was strewn with newspapers, pens, papers and an open dictionary. Although he relished this time to himself, we all knew he hadn't wanted to step down from work, but certain changes in him meant he simply could not continue. For a while now he had seemed . . . like a different, disconnected, distant Dad. The man who brought power to so many had become powerless, his light slowly dimming at the end of his performance.

At some point the cared-for become the carers. This is true whether you have children or pets or loved ones. The only way to avoid this is to live alone in the wilderness. So we end up having to care for the people who once cared for us; this isn't a shame and it isn't a tragedy and it isn't a chore. It is an honour. To be able to return the gift of love that someone bestows upon you is a gift in itself.

This is a story of caring . . .

# My Mad Dad

## *17th August*

Today I started a new life. In many ways it's a return to my old one, but so much has changed. This morning I woke up in my bedroom in small-town Pontypool, South Wales. Yesterday, I came round to the buzzing of busy traffic outside my Camden studio flat – the home of drunk noise. Several friends were asleep on the sofa and floor, alongside empty bottles of cheap vodka, cartons of cigarettes and a broken Sex Pistols CD. This morning, my cohabitants included one mentally ill parent, a bumper-sized packet of Ibuprofen, information on senile dementia and a Cliff Richard *Greatest Hits* CD.

I left my flat when most of the others were still passed out. One rogue hand managed to peek out from under a duvet and bid me farewell. I zipped up my favourite Rick Owens leather jacket and slung my large travel bag containing the last of my London possessions – a few band T-shirts, fancy cosmetics gifted to me from industry parties, my diary and a pen – over my shoulder and closed the door on the small studio apartment that had defined me for so long. That final click of a life less ordinary, the excitement I sought, my escape route from the valleys and my ticket to independence was now due its return journey.

It was the end of an era in more ways than one. Saying goodbye to this life also meant finally saying goodbye to that part of my life I shared with him. The ex who I'd thought was the one. While still raw, our split is only a small part of my troubles right now. I've got bigger things to worry about than trying to dance with someone who doesn't want to dance with me.

The dull grey of a muggy north London morning was still bright enough to warrant sunglasses, or perhaps it was just my straining eyes and lack of sleep. Nodding familiarly at market traders setting up for the day, I stopped at the newsagent for cigarettes and soft drinks and noticed some kids buying booze for their 11am come-downs after a long night of clubbing. I strode across the busy streets, swerving through pedestrians and vehicles, and made for the bus. I rode the almost-empty 27 bus all the way from Camden Town to Paddington, clutching onto a carton of hangover-quelling Ribena for dear life and taking the best seat in the house – top deck, front right. I love peering into people's houses and apartments, into gardens and shops. The hum of NW1 seldom rests: punks still smoking on the lock bridge – no sleep for them – pubs cleaning up after another night's fun, undercover police not being that undercover around the tube station. The whole place just makes me smile.

Eventually the bus cut along the bottom of Regent's Park and past the already lengthy queues of tourists outside Madame Tussauds, and trundled over Edgware Road towards Paddington Station. Fumbling half-heartedly for my seldom-cleared credit card to pay for my extortionately priced ticket, I strode through the din towards the Cardiff-bound train and settled into my stained seat.

I was half dozing off before we'd even pulled out of the station, that surreal half-wake when you're only just aware of your surroundings and pretty power-less over them. I was leaving the city behind just as it was warming up. Passing towns got smaller, first Reading then Swindon; fields and farms sped by, the long thick train powering in and out of tunnels that carve up patchwork England. My eyes grew heavier and my mobile-phone signal dim. I changed lines just over the Welsh border at Newport and took a smaller train up to the valleys, to Pontypool. It didn't take long; I stood for the journey, my face leaning out of the vestibule window, warm Welsh air blowing my dirty blonde, cigarette-scented hair on and off my face. The colours seemed bolder, deeper-green hues all around, and the smell was subtle and sweet; no take-away grease, no beer-stained pavements, no buses honking their dissatisfaction at insolent pedestrians. Just small-town life, quiet and gentle, safe and soft.

The train station at Pontypool and New Inn is so small it is unmanned. There isn't a ticket booth or machine, no gates – nothing – just some concrete in the middle of nowhere. We used to come here to smoke and drink as teenagers – one of our many haunts – but now it feels more vast and lonely than ever. Unsurprisingly, I was the only person to alight at this station; very often you have to find the driver and actually request the stop, like a bloody bus or something. My booted feet landed heavy on the platform and seemed to echo a warning, but there was no one there to heed that, only me.

The house is more than a mile and a half from the station and is an uphill climb. I ambled past the homes of my childhood friends; my old junior school; the pub and post office; the streets where I'd learned to ride my bike; the eerie cemetery we used to run past for no reason other than it was a cemetery and we were kids; the garages behind which I'd had my first cigarette, my first swig of cider, my first kiss. It seemed much quieter this afternoon and smaller, muted and subdued, tired and old. This was the town where my memories had been made. The town that made me, for better or worse, the person I am now, the returned. Nothing was the same, yet nothing had changed. Except me.

The hill to the house is a real fucker, steep and sharp; even in a car you struggle, exhaust choking and engine revving, but the view from the top is spectacular. I climbed steeply, leaning into the camber, sweating pure alcohol into my leather jacket and breathing hard. The pale sunshine had burned through the clouds and the afternoon was becoming warm, well, warm for Wales at least. I got a few waves from people in shops that I passed, old acquaintances, a beep from a passing car driven by an old neighbour flapping a hand furiously out of the window, a smile from a lady in her front yard hanging out her washing, and I took it all in, this being 'home'.

As I reached the gate posts, I turned to look over the town, propping up my breathless carcass with one hand on the wrought-iron gate. I was looking out over rooftops again but, unlike London, there was more space, it was greener, and the town seemed to smile more. It was less exciting, certainly, but less risky, too, more manageable. There are no strangers here, everyone knows everyone – for better or worse. These people know me and they know my family. There was a certain poignancy to the song playing through my headphones. It was 'Old Man' by Neil Young.

'Hello, Mammy,' I called out as I sneaked through the door, which my parents rarely keep locked – it's a small-town thing.

'Och, love! We weren't expecting you until tomorrow!' Mum cried, her gentle and subtle Scots lilt taking me back to her reading nursery rhymes to me as a wee nipper. She looked genuinely shocked to see me. Rising slowly from the battered, old, brown leather sofa (older than Gareth and me), she swayed towards me in the doorway in classic Mum uniform: long, floral-patterned, linen Marks & Spencer skirt and a crinkled cotton cardigan in pastel shades of lilac, iris and mauve. She clutched me close to her and stroked my hair, the way mums do.

'I'm so pleased you're here,' she added, her perfume and hairspray sticking fast in my throat and making me feel like a child again, happy, warm and safe.

'Where's Da?'

'Out in the shed, love. I'm not sure why, but he's OK.'

'Is he?' I found that hard to believe, however much I wanted to.

'Yeah . . . yeah,' she replied unconvincingly. (Mental note – must work on hiding my sarcastic tone of voice.)

I have returned to Wales to help Mum look after Dad, who is very ill with Alzheimer's. He was diagnosed a year ago, and as my parents are getting older and Dad's behaviour is causing concern among our family and friends, I have come back to lend a helping hand. I decided to resign from my job as an assistant fashion buyer for a London department store only a matter of weeks ago. If I'm honest, although I'm only 25, I had become rather tired of it all and when Dad became ill, I found little comfort in the shallow, artificial world of fashion. Perhaps others would have sought shelter in the 'importance' of the next big trend in fall/winter shades of red, but I knew there were far bigger issues lurking and I couldn't hide away and use my career as an avoidance tactic. Saying that, I'd not wanted to quit my life in London for anything; I value my independence and I love carving out a life all of my own, but the dynamics of that existence had also started to change – and not really for the better. Maybe a bit of 'time out' will do me good, though I think a year's trip around Indonesia would be more enjoyable than returning home to look after ageing parents.

While in London I had managed to avoid thinking too much about my impending return to Wales, as I didn't want to upset myself. I was in denial, I suppose. In the same manner, I will try to avoid thinking of London too much while I'm here. Yet as each hour passes I miss it more than I thought possible and the slow, dawning realisation of what lies ahead does, quite frankly, freak me out.

I had a much-needed shower while Mum made us all tea. I felt like a whole new human already, washing the day-old stench of a hangover away, rinsing the last of my London life off my skin and down the plughole, and taking comfort in the smell of the shower gel my family have used since the dawn of time. Chucking on some old clothes, I came back downstairs to see Dad emerging from the shed, bringing some old chains wrapped in newspaper to 'look at and figure out'. He looked as he usually did, a little paler perhaps, a little greyer – they both did

– smaller and less vivid, just like the old home town. He had come in from the garden as the afternoon sun faded; we'd left him to his own devices until then, just Mum and I chatting around the issues but never confronting them. I wanted to leave him be for now, to delay the inevitable, but when he finally trundled up the garden path and in through the old lean-to, stomping the dirt from his feet, he didn't seem to think me being home was a big deal. We hadn't seen each other in about three months but that didn't register, for him.

'Hello, my love,' he cooed, as if I were a toddler, taking my shoulders firmly and lovingly in each large hand and kissing me on the forehead. He had grease and woodchip on his polo shirt and down his cords; he loved being in that shed, it gave him a sense of purpose. Perhaps it made him think or feel that he was still working, as if he was still worth something. I don't know if he realises that this is a full-time thing, me being home. I'm guessing not. He asked me how university was and after a quick sideways glance to a sighing Mum, I told him it was fine. He set about washing his hands from his 'work', telling us that he has really progressed with the project, and then washed his hands again. I was about to tell him he'd done it once, but Mum just shook her head, an indication that this was just one of many things we were to let go.

After a dinner of chicken and salad round our old dining table we settled down to watch some telly, but I was so tired I went to bed at 8pm, falling right to sleep. The peace, the quiet, the clean bed, the fresh linen and the comfort were womb-like. My hangover had numbed my emotions. The sick feeling, as a result of too many sambucas, had taken command of my senses, allowing no room for emotional distress or wistful melancholy for the existence I was leaving behind, which was definitely a blessing in disguise. However, I am still aware of it being far too quiet here. I know I was raised here, like this, but I've become used to something else. Almost every night for the past four years I've fallen asleep to the sounds of pubs chucking out their last customers, of trains, buses, police sirens and general city din. I find this return to a void of sound most unsettling. The quiet of the countryside gives me the willies. I know that people think you get nutters in big cities, and it's true – I happen to know many of them – but I have always been of the opinion that the most dangerous madmen would choose to inhabit quieter rural idylls. Out here, no one can hear you scream.

With that thought, I went to sleep and dreamed of London. I dreamed about my friends all sitting in our pub in Camden, The Good Mixer, drinking and laughing. I couldn't hear what they were saying, but I could see their lips moving in vivid conversation. I wished I could pick up the gist. I was merely a spectator in their evening. They couldn't see me and that was upsetting; my life was going on without me.

## *18th August*

I awoke this morning to the sound of heavy rain, which is a huge part of life in the South Wales valleys. Even in summer, it's a constant that you can always rely on. To some extent, I had forgotten just how beautiful and vast the landscape is here. With my nose pressed up against the glass of my bedroom window, I sat and watched sheets of rain fall quickly over the mountains. The town below in the hollow of the valley was completely obscured from sight. You could have been forgiven for assuming that there was nothing there, and it looked as if someone had just filled the valley with grey, soggy cotton wool.

On a clear day (not like today, which is all grey and overcast) you can see for miles and miles from here, right over the Severn to Bristol and down to the Somerset coast. It's nothing like London, where you can't see past the end of the street. The town at the bottom of the hill is very small but much has changed since I left. A Tesco supermarket has been built and this really is progress gone mad! There is also a Wetherspoons pub, which my dad was most taken with for a while before he stopped being able to go out on his own. Well, we at least try to discourage him from doing this; the problem with dementia is that once it hits a certain point, the sufferer seldom thinks there is anything wrong with them, and my dad is a very proud man. He also likes visiting pubs.

My breath steamed up the glass and after I had written my initials in the misty covering I went downstairs. The house is very traditional; a Victorian semi with a small yard to the front and a lovely little garden to the back. My mum has kept it pretty much as it was when my brother and I left all those years ago. Our bedrooms are almost like shrines to us. Teddy bears still rest on our pillows, their bodies tucked under the duvets. Sports-day medals and gymkhana rosettes adorn the walls and school photos and swimming badges are proudly displayed on bedside tables that are dusted daily. Perhaps on some level my parents knew we would return, and that even though it might take years and may not be under the most pleasant of circumstances, it was still worth refraining from changing anything. Had they been waiting for us to return, or had they never really accepted that we had left?

Mum wanted to go to Tesco, so I offered to help her with the shopping – she isn't as strong as she used to be these days. I suppose that's just what happens when you get old, although at 61 she's hardly an OAP and still works full-time for the charity. As an office administrator, I think she is probably the most under-titled person ever; I'm pretty sure she kind of runs the show. She's one of those people you just ask for anything and everything because she knows how/where/why/when/whom. I bet 'Dunno, ask Marge' is one of the most commonly used phrases in her office.

When we left the house, we told Dad not to go out, but we held little hope of him actually following our instructions. The best we could hope for was that the rain would keep him housebound for a while at least.

When we returned from the shops, he was, to our surprise, still about, but the house reeked of burning.

'Burned the toast, have you, Dad?' I asked.

He looked up blankly from the dining table, coffee mug in hand and glasses on nose.

'Uh?' he replied, following a long pause.

'I said it smells of burned toast. Have you had your breakfast then, yeah?'

'Yeah, oh yeah. I like my breakfast I do. It's nice. I had toast, love.'

'Good, good. You've got your jumper on back to front by the way.'

'Ah, fuck off.'

'Don't speak to your daughter like that!' Mum snapped, looking shocked even though this language was a more frequent occurrence these days.

'You can fuck off, too,' he added for good measure.

I didn't know whether to laugh or be offended; I mean, I am pretty used to foul language, I'm a big fan of it personally, but when I saw Dad's shoulders shaking I knew he was laughing. I laughed along, too, but Mum was miffed, and left the room. Dad didn't usually use the F word – it was a more recent addition to his vocabulary. I don't know whether it was intentional, accidental, par for the course or just an excuse to speak his mind while he still had it.

Sometimes it isn't really worth talking to Dad. I don't mean that in a bad way, although I know it sounds really terrible and I'm aware that I am taking a negative tone with him today, as I am still a bit tired and grumpy about everything. But even Mum is very short with him these days. The only person Dad listens to is Gareth. Dad loves my brother. In fact, everyone loves my brother. If my mum or I ask Dad to do something he gets very insulted and becomes aggressive and defensive. On the other hand, if it comes from Gareth he obediently obliges with the utmost care and respect. It must be a male thing. Either that or he really doesn't like my mum. Or me.

I can hear a song by the Smashing Pumpkins playing on a radio somewhere. I have avoided listening to music as I know every song will remind me of London and will risk triggering a massive crying session. I don't want to do that. I want to almost ignore these feelings until they dilute themselves and become little more than rose-tinted nostalgia. I've only been home a couple of days and I am already massively missing my friends, but I truly believe this is the best way to deal with a situation that has practically been forced upon me by circumstances way beyond anyone's control. It no longer matters if I am upset, there are far bigger issues at stake.

This afternoon, my mum is going to the local prison to serve tea to inmates and their visiting families and friends. She is very kind like that. She does this every other Saturday and is on a rota with other ladies in the community, who do similarly kind and selfless deeds for other people. As a result, it's just Dad and me in the house. Right now, he is downstairs waiting for the rugby game to come on the telly. I shall probably go down and join him in a bit. I think he would like the company and, to be honest, so would I. There isn't much scope for companionship this weekend, so I guess it's just me and him; the stranger I have known for 25 years.

## 19th August

As I sit down to write this today, I am eating the leftovers of the fish pie I made for Mum and Dad last night. I thought that I was quite a good chef, but Mum said that I hadn't cooked the pastry for long enough. She is very good in the kitchen, though, so I take the feedback on the chin. Dad enjoyed it, though he hasn't been much of a barometer of taste these days. Everything he eats seems to be the best thing he has ever tasted and he constantly remarks on how wonderful his food is. Right now, he seems to be totally enamoured with small pots of desserts, such as trifles or chocolate mousses.

'Oh, these things are wonderful, aren't they, love?' he'll remark to Mum, usually more than once, over the course of devouring one. 'Just all in one little pot – marvellous.'

He is also rather taken with muffins and cakes, which is strange, as when we were growing up I don't ever recall him having much of a sweet tooth. I'm aware that sometimes Alzheimer's brings about changes in the sufferer's personality, but gastronomic tastes? I must look it up.

'Cor, I do love these little cakey things,' he said to me earlier, 'and you can get them anywhere now. The Tesco, the market, the Greggs bakers. I think I've even seen them in the little shop on the corner – and I've seen them in the Tesco, too.'

Often Dad forgets he's eaten one and has about three in a night. Though I'm not sure if he really is forgetting . . .

I dreamed about London again last night. I have a feeling this is going to be a recurrent part of my non-waking life, at least for a while. It was London again, except it didn't look like London. You know the way that sometimes happens in dreams? You feel that you are in a certain place, yet it looks completely different. In the dream, I wandered around Camden and said a quick but silent farewell to my favourite shops, bars, cafés and restaurants. This is something I'd avoided doing during my last few days there, probably for fear of getting too upset. I regret that now, as I am starting to wonder when, if ever, I will return and how much things might change in the meantime.

The mundane routine of life here is falling around me like some sort of drab, heavy cloak and I have an inkling that I will not be able to shed it for a very long time. It's all right for my dad – every day is a brand new adventure for him.

My mum woke me this morning at 7:45. She was bored and had been up very early, which she seems to be doing a lot of lately. Perhaps I should ask why she isn't sleeping well? It must have something to do with the fact that she's lying next to Dad, who apparently snores like a freight train and kicks around in his sleep like Michael Flatley.

I went downstairs to make some breakfast, mixing together some berries and yoghurt. I have made the decision to go on a health kick. My supermarket trips no longer comprise value and orange-sticker goods and seeing which spirits are on special offer. I've vowed to give up the fags and get myself a bit fitter, too. I'm the first to admit I haven't been leading much of a healthy lifestyle of late; too much booze, partying and late nights. I guess it's only when you step outside your friendship circle that you realise your old ways weren't as 'normal' as you initially thought. They only appeared that way because they were what everyone else was doing. Perhaps that's why we all hung around together – we made each other feel normal. We knew we could get as wasted as we wanted and no one would judge us because we were all the same. Did we all really delude ourselves into thinking we were good friends? Would we have hung out together so much if we weren't all so focused on partying? Would putting a stop to all the drinking mean I would spend less time with them? Our recreational habits went hand in hand with a certain element of selfishness and I couldn't help but wonder who out of my friends would actually be there for me if the going got really tough. I have a feeling I am about to find out.

This afternoon my mum is going to a barbecue at her friend's house. She has a really good group of mates and they all support each other and do lots of fun things like hill walking, outdoor pursuits and keeping fit – they even share an allotment. I know my mum has not been able to do so much with them recently, and I am glad I'm here to help look after Dad so that she can have a bit of her life back. I hope I have friends like hers when I'm older. My dad doesn't really have mates any more. I think he has become alienated and marginalised, and this makes me very sad. I don't want to think of him as lonely.

## 21st August

Last night I went to a party at my best friend Ellie's. I've known her since I was nine and she lives in Cardiff now. Many school friends have migrated there; it's only about 40 minutes from the house and is a nice buzzing city, especially in comparison to sleepy little Pontypool.

It was good to get out of the house for a while and escape my parents. It was also nice to meet up with some old friends that I haven't seen in a long time. I'm touched by the generosity of some folk, especially of those I haven't had much to do with for many years. Around here, old friendships aren't quickly forgotten. I finally managed to get a charger for my phone (I left the last one in the flat) and called a few friends in London. Their first reaction was to yell at me for leaving the pub early and going back to the flat without saying goodbye. I thought this was a little short-sighted and insensitive on their part. The reason I left before bidding them farewell was because I was massively upset about the turn my life was taking . . . not that I have to justify my actions to anyone. If they feel all they can do in life is stay out late every night just to avoid their personal issues then that's their problem. I've got enough to deal with to be bothered by this sort of trivial shit.

When I got in last night, Mum and Dad were watching telly. Dad wasn't really watching, rather he was just staring blankly into space – arms folded tightly across his chest and in another world. He has a volunteer carer who takes him out every Monday morning, a lovely lady who lives locally. They mainly do the same thing each week (not that my dad would notice) and I wonder if he behaves as bizarrely with her as he does with Mum and me. I think they just go into town and walk around for a while. She must listen to him jabber on like a monkey in a tree, and he must enjoy having someone new to jabber on to.

God knows that Mum and I don't really listen any more. I feel awful for saying this, but sometimes I can't bear it. I must be the most selfish and horrible girl in the whole world. Perhaps I wouldn't find it so bad if this was happening to someone else. It's just that it's my dad and I want to shake him, scream at the top of my voice and tell him that I just want him to BE NORMAL.

I heard an analogy the other day; it was on the telly, I think, and a spokesperson compared the early stages of Alzheimer's disease to a radio that tuned in and out, sometimes working, sometimes very clear and sometimes just fuzzy, completely impossible to decipher or understand. I try to keep that in mind with Dad, but it isn't easy. It makes me livid to think that his brilliant mind is now not so brilliant. And why? Because of some weak genetics? Some pointless degeneration? Something has stolen the most brilliant part of this man.

I'm thinking of doing some volunteer work with other local people who suffer from dementia. I reckon I would be able to deal with it if it just wasn't so close to home and the person I was helping was someone else and not my dad. I also think that it would be good in some kind of karmic way. If I can't really look after my dad then perhaps I could do it for someone else. Maybe then things in the universe would somehow retain their balance, as I would still be contributing to the good deeds in the world. I hope that's the way things work out.

In the afternoon, I had a row with Dad. Mum had a doctor's appointment and he was just meandering around the house. I had asked him to do something to help me (I can't even remember what it was now, shut a door or something), and he turned really nasty really quickly.

'Why don't you just fuck off? Go on – no one wants you here,' he yelled, his face snarling and strange, as though it belonged to another man and not my dad.

I was furious and shouted back: 'Don't want me here? Well, who the fuck is going to look after you then, eh?'

'Look after me? I don't need looking after, you petulant little shit. There's nothing wrong with me!'

'Nothing wrong with you? Dad, you're terminally ill, you're fucking nuts!'

'I am? Me?' he yelled back indignantly. He truly didn't understand that there was anything wrong with him and he thought I was just talking shit.

'Dad, you've got Alzheimer's!' I wailed helplessly. He just stared blankly in response, the pause button hit on his brain.

We both just stared into the moment, me deeply regretting losing my cool but angry that Dad didn't realise or appreciate that people were trying to help him. Then I felt more regret for not appreciating that he really didn't know. He couldn't help his actions, but I could help mine, or at least I should.

This is the first time he's forgotten he is ill. Up until now he has always been fairly philosophical about the impact of his illness, saying that he was lucky to have had such a good life and that the disease was not impinging on his day-to-day activities – he was just a little forgetful. I stormed out, as he blatantly didn't understand any more and we were just upsetting each other. I wanted to cry so badly, but I refused to let myself.

Instead, I went to the local leisure centre for a swim. It's the same one I used to go to as a child. I remember when they opened a new section with slides and everything, the whole town went mad for it, it could possibly have been the best thing that happened to Pontypool that year! It has undergone a bit of a makeover since then but it still has its faded old tiled murals on the pool walls, the plastic stadium seating laid empty to the side and the squash courts smelling of the early 1990s. And it still only cost £2 for a swim – £2! I did 10 lengths, as it's a big pool. Slipping into the lukewarm, over-chlorinated water felt like a cleansing baptism, purging me of my short-tempered slurs and poor care skills. With every swing of my arms and kick of my legs I felt freer and stronger.

Now, I'm a lot better for it, although it's made me realise how unfit I am. My chest still burns like a raging bush fire, and my calf muscles are aching and I already know that tomorrow it will be worse. But I am trying, I am trying to be stronger. I am determined to use my time here well in many ways; I hate the notion of wasted time and while looking after someone is never time wasted, I feel as if trans-formation of self is also needed.

After I finished my punishing swim I floated around in the deep end, the sounds muffled by the thick water, everything feeling far away and muted. I feel stuck in limbo. Most of my possessions are still scattered around a few friends' houses in London, and without my stuff here I can't really call it 'home'. It just doesn't feel like it. I feel like I'm nowhere.

## 22nd August

Dad is being nice today. I woke late, went downstairs and when I softly padded into the sitting room in my slippered feet, he told me how nice I looked. This was a bit odd considering I hadn't even cleaned my face, brushed my teeth or washed my hair. Perhaps that is how his illness makes him see things now, in their purest, most unadulterated form. Or perhaps he was trying to make amends for telling me that I had a big nose last night (this is true – I do have a big nose), although he's probably well past the stage of even attempting to make amends now. He doesn't remember his misdemeanours.

There was the most beautiful sunset here last night. I had forgotten how stunning they can be during my years in London – out here you can see so much more sky. The sun was being forced down behind the mountains, as if it was trying desperately to stay out and play long after its bedtime. It tarnished the underbelly of the clouds a riotous amber, in childish defiance of its imposed curfew, while the top of the clouds were tinged authoritarian indigo – maintaining that it was high time the sun went to bed. I was watching all this play out from my bedroom window, sitting on the floor with my chin resting on hands folded over the windowsill, the final streams of sunlight causing me to squint. Peace and nature were interrupted when I suddenly remembered I hadn't given Dad his evening medicine, so I ran back downstairs. By the time I had managed to coerce him into taking his pills (by agreeing with him that they were in fact Viagra and wasn't that very funny?) and raced back upstairs to my window-side resting spot, fingermarks still on the glass, the sun had well and truly set. The sky had taken on a darkening lilac colour and there was no more to see – the night was coming in.

## 23rd August

Today I went with Mum to an Alzheimer's Society carers' meeting. The local community seems to accommodate support groups very well and there is a wealth of advice and help at hand. The meeting was held in a bright and well-worn room with pale olive, patterned curtains, an old, dark blue, ridged carpet with chewing-gum stains, and a telly in the corner dated circa 1979. The attendees arrived thick and fast, and as I was the youngest there by about 30 years I helped to pass out the chairs. Mum was feeling quite weak  again, the strain of looking after Dad was clearly taking its toll.  I wondered if she was ill, but Mum never gets ill.

The crowd was exactly as I had imagined; mostly ladies of a certain age caring for their husbands. Their men had stood by them through decades of marriage, but sadly their minds had not made the journey. I felt a little awkward and out of place; like a fraud or an imposter. I wished I were one. Out of about 15 people, only three were men; one was caring for his mother and was flanked by his sister and wife, who shared the duties. They had obviously convinced him to come along, as he didn't look too comfortable.

The second man was the sole carer for his wife and the third had been part of the carers' group for some years but had lost his wife to Alzheimer's very recently. I immediately asked myself why he was there. This group was for carers and he didn't fall into that category any more. My mum later explained that if you look after someone full-time, when they eventually go it can leave an even bigger hole in your life than it would have done had they not been ill. That man's entire life had been devoted to caring for his wife and now that she was gone it was likely he had nothing that would fill the vacant hours of his day. The group had kept him going for so long.

They had been his forum, his voice and, very often I suspect, his escape. It was his chance to talk to someone and to have his say. Whatever he said at home to his wife would have fallen on deaf ears. Perhaps attending the Alzheimer's support meetings kept her memory alive; this was a part of his life that he was not ready to let go of yet.

My mum also said that he might have wanted to pass on his advice to others who were still dealing with what he had endured. He seemed a very lovely gentleman, kind of like a local grandpa, smartly turned out, the little hair he had left gelled subtly to one side of his round, friendly face. He gently cleared his throat every time before he spoke and I listened intently to what he said. He told the group how he had been feeling this week, since their last meeting, although I highly suspect that what he said was carefully constructed and rehearsed. He said that he felt a little better this week. That he had finally got around to going through some of his wife's clothes, thinking about what best to do with them. He had bought new bed sheets and had found this very hard because this was the first thing that was now just his. Not his and hers. A symbolic 'moving on'. I could tell that he was about to cry as he stopped talking, looked at his feet, and cleared his throat again. When we got home I burst into tears. I cried because I was glad to see my dad (even though he hadn't noticed that we had even gone out), but I also cried because that man must have gone home to an empty house that still smelled of his wife. I had people around me to take my mind off my tears (Dad just talked about his shoes and Mum watched *Poirot*), and I hoped that the man wasn't too lonely and that he too had someone, somewhere.

The meeting made me question why there were so few men present. I'd done my research and knew that Alzheimer's isn't a gender-discriminatory disease. I wondered whether perhaps it was an issue of pride and also maybe a generational thing. Us women are better talkers, aren't we? My mum and aunt certainly seemed to prove this theory. Are women more likely to seek out a support group than men? In this day and age are we not more inclined to admit to having problems where mental health is concerned? I feel compelled to lessen the negative stigma attached to so-called 'embarrassing' illnesses but I don't know how. Maybe writing this diary will help, even if it is only for my benefit.

There were also a few ladies at the group whose husbands had gone into care. Their stories are inescapably sad and they made me think about having to put Dad into full-time care one day. This would entail admitting that I wasn't up to the job, that I couldn't care for him any more and that I was going to have to give up. The ladies mentioned that their partners actually quite liked living in care, and when they were taken out for the day they often asked to go home – not to the homes they shared with their wives, but to the only place they now knew. The nests the women had feathered for their husbands were now unrecognisable to them – unwanted almost, ungratefully redundant. One lady said that the hardest part of living on her own after her husband had gone into care was cooking for one. She told me how she had put on weight, not through comfort eating but because, after decades of cooking every meal for two, she was unable to prepare meals only for herself. I think the weight gain provided the comfort necessary to eclipse the pain of eating alone and the ignominy of buying meals for one.

## 24th August

I had forgotten what living in a small town is like. In many circumstances, it's quite nice and it's most certainly the best place to be if you have some sort of illness. People are far kinder and more accommodating – it is a far more sedentary pace of life. Buses drive slower and the drivers wave at each other. People say hello to strangers in the street. Dog walkers stop to let you pat their pets and the girls at the supermarket checkout make small talk with real sincerity. The lady at the counter in the bank enquires after your mum and the man in the corner shop lets you off the five pence you are short of for a pint of milk. He says he'll 'get it next time', with a wink and a smile. I'm yet to fully immerse myself in this way of life and I'm hoping I won't have to, but it's still comforting to know that this kind of behaviour is prevalent across the country. Not everyone is a grumpy, busy Londoner like me!

My skin is beginning to look different and I think I have lost a few pounds. I am sleeping for at least eight hours a night and the tap water tastes far superior to what London has to offer from its dirty faucets. The other night I even bought a gin and tonic for £1.50. I was truly shocked, and also impressed.

The truth is, though, I am still bored. I've only been gone a week and already I miss my friends and my old life. I miss my independence. I need to get my driver's licence and then I will be as free as a bird (who drives her mother's car and can't go too far away . . . ).

## 25th August

I started to think last night about how my dad must be feeling now. When he was first diagnosed with Alzheimer's at the age of 60, he just sat there and didn't comment. It was our mum who told us, following a meal at a hotel. It wasn't really a surprise, as I think we had all known for some time – Dad included. He'd told my brother and me the previous summer that he felt like he was losing his mind. He said he wanted to let us know before he went properly insane and started talking to walls – which subsequently did happen. It was nice of him to have given us a warning, I thought.

That weekend, about two years ago, I had taken a train from London to a hotel in the Home Counties, where my brother was working. Mum and Dad had been staying there for the weekend and thought it would be nice if we all got together for supper on the Saturday night. We had a nice evening and were commenting on how good the meal had been, when my mum said she wanted to make an announcement.

'We have something to tell you,' she began, barely looking up from the table. 'Your father has been diagnosed with Alzheimer's disease.'

I could still taste my beef Wellington. I thought I was about to choke.

Dad looked at his empty plate and made no eye contact with us at all. I wasn't shocked, as we'd all suspected that this was coming, but I did feel sick – this was now a reality. Those words were out there now. *This was happening.*

When the whole 'diagnosis' thing was revealed that evening, my mum also dropped in another gem of information. My dad was adopted. Now, I had always thought that he was Welsh through and through, born and bred. It turns out this wasn't the case. Apparently, Dad was born in London during the Blitz and was only a small baby when he was sent to live in Wales, away from the bombings in the capital and all other horrible things associated with war that children should never have to witness. Some distant relatives in the Rhondda Valley took him in. It was real coal-mining country – that's what almost everyone did back then, and his family were no different. They were the typical no-frills, 'tin bath in front of the fire every Sunday' types whose children never spoke. Not that anyone seemed to mind, as far as I know; Dad always spoke pleasantly about his early life. I guess he never really knew what happened to his biological parents, or even whether they survived the war. He referred to the people who raised him as his mum and dad. Dad has three older 'sisters' and, from what I can gather, he was a happy little boy. As a family, we were always closer to my mum's side, who are Scottish, and it had seemed strange to me that we never really saw much of Dad's clan, even though they only lived on the other side of Cardiff. By the same token, we would drive up to spend summers and Christmases in Scotland. Now I knew the reason for this – they weren't really 'family', if we're being technical about it. This just added to the smack-in-the-face feeling you are left with after you have been told that your father is mentally on a downhill slope towards total insanity. This point now strikes me with increased resonance; Dad is having trouble recognising himself now, but in so many respects perhaps he never really knew who he was.

Dad's diagnosis hit my brother harder than me. After Mum and Dad had gone to bed, G and I stayed up at the bar and had a drink. He was angry and tearful, furious at why this had happened to us, why Dad? I'm not emotionally stunted, but I just couldn't see the point of crying about it. What good would it do? Besides, this disease is indiscriminate, so if not us then why anyone? Why does anyone get old and ill and die? That's just what happens in life. Maybe G thought that as the older sibling he would have to carry more of the strain than me. Maybe I wasn't getting it.

Anyway, nothing much happened after that. I went back to London, Mum and Dad went back to Wales and my brother went back to work. Sounds a bit blasé, I know, but that's what happened. We get it from our parents, always playing things down. Maybe it did affect me more than I let myself realise. I got smashed in the pub the next afternoon with some friends. Looking back, I was trying to numb myself some more, not wanting, not ready, not able to deal with it.

### 28th August

Today I thought about how, in hindsight, there had been some tell-tale signs of Dad's illness that I only recognise now. Things at the time seemed just a bit odd, but I put that down to the old man mellowing with age – I certainly never thought he was ill. I also don't really like to use the term 'ill', because apart from the obvious mental block, my dad remains as fit as a fiddle. However, I suppose it is an illness and even though he would hate to be referred to as poorly, I shall refer to him as so.

I remember coming home from university one dark winter's evening before he got ill. Mum was out and I could tell Dad was pleased to see me, which was nice, especially as he was always kind of cantankerous while I was growing up. He gave me a hug and started jabbering on about how good the train service was between Wales and London. It was a speech I'd heard a thousand times before, but one I had to agree with nevertheless. He helped me with my bags, which wasn't a rarity as he was always very manly in that respect. If something needed lifting, Dad was your man! Then we went into the kitchen and he asked me if I was hungry.

'Dad, I'm a student, of course I'm hungry. I'm always hungry!' I replied.

'Well,' he said excitedly. 'I thought you might like some eggs or something. Look, I've got the frying pan out and I've even put a bit of oil in it, so it's all ready for you.'

True to his word, Dad had done all this for me. He smiled with satisfaction, hands on hips and chest out proud.

'Eh, thanks, Dad,' I replied, a little bemused. 'Just what I wanted!'

It wasn't, incidentally. I had a foul hangover and the last thing I wanted was fried eggs. Despite this, I proceeded to cook myself some with Dad's enthusiastic assistance. He duly provided support in such crucial tasks as passing the butter for the toast and getting a plate out, and so on. Then we sat and talked while I ate. Well, he talked really, and I just nodded occasionally and thought about how weird it was that my non-domesticated father had readied a pan of oil for his hungry daughter's return from university. Sweet, but weird. As I've said, this was before his diagnosis, so I thought little more about it. I just assumed he was growing into a more chilled and less grumpy person. He looked happy that he had provided the necessary refreshment for his offspring, but that is what parents need to feel, I guess. They need to feel that they have provided – men especially. And my dad did provide.

In fact, my dad was great; although I haven't always thought so. Children go through phases of liking their parents, and often these phases directly correlate to how many presents they get, how late they are allowed to stay up at weekends and how embarrassing those parents were when dancing at their 11th birthday party. However, that aside, my dad was pretty good, as dads go. I didn't grow up with any of the horror stories of abuse, neglect or broken homes. My childhood was fairly idyllic. While I didn't recall thinking they were all that great at the time, I have always had huge respect for my parents; we never went without – in fact, we had more than enough. Although I can't always pinpoint the dates for his departure for foreign postings and subsequent reappearance in our lives, I do recall 'missing' Dad when he worked away. That said, I had friends who saw less of their fathers who lived with them. One of my friend's dads worked at a local factory, making car brake parts or something. He would have to work nightshifts, so any time I went round hers to play after school he would be asleep on the sofa. At the time, I didn't really understand why and just thought he was lazy!

So while I did feel a little envious of my friends who saw their dads whenever they wanted, anything to do with my dad was always exciting. Going for really long trips on aeroplanes, being somewhere hot with a swimming pool, eating new foods and seeing crazy things. One year we had to go to China for the whole summer, and I remember seeing the Terracotta Army and some mummified woman who still had her hair even though her body was reputed to be thousands of years old. Dad took us round some factory he had set up, which smelled so strongly of jasmine, and people all stopped working to bow their heads when he walked past.

One night, a banquet was held in his honour, and we all had to put on smart clothes and got driven there in a fancy car. As is apparently customary in that area, a fish head was brought out of the kitchen and placed in front of my mum for her delectation. She nearly retched at the sight of it, all bulging eyes and leaky brains. As she stood to give faux thanks to the clapping dinner attendees, she wondered how on earth she could get away with not eating it. Before she could muster some sort of crap about not eating fish, she looked down to see my brother, chopsticks in hand, going to town on the macabre dish of honour. My dad stood up and proudly declared, 'That's my boy!' The evening was too long and I fell asleep in my chair. It was raining and stormy outside and the staff arranged for our car to collect us and take us home. I have vague recollections of Dad scooping me up in his arms and carrying me out of the hotel via the back way, through the less-than-salubrious kitchens and galleys to our waiting car. The rain hammered heavily on the old tin roof, but he had us safe.

## 29th August

Alzheimer's is a very variable disease, as are all associated forms of dementia, so I have learned. Sometimes it can progress very quickly and sometimes sufferers can go on for years displaying very few advancing symptoms. I remember being at a doctor's appointment with Mum and Dad at some point after his diagnosis (mainly to support Mum). The doctor told us, with some joy, that the chances were he would die of something totally unrelated to his disease, such as cancer, or even a car crash! Nice. It seems that Dad is falling into the first category of progression. Obviously, following the diagnosis, we began to attribute all his bizarre behaviour to the disease. Repetition of stories has undoubtedly become more frequent, but he has also started to make things up. Now, my dad has always been one for spinning a good yarn, and embellishment is fine for the sake of a good story, however, now that it's apparent that his memories have all but up and left him, I think he has started to create new ones to replace the ones that have fled his ageing mind. The 'untruths' vary in eminence from 'Yes, I've taken my medicine' to 'Ooh, I had fish for tea'. As I write, I can hear my mum muttering in the background, 'Chicken, darling, it was chicken.' These days it is becoming harder to decipher what he has actually done and what he has made up.

I guess the earliest stages of the disease hit Dad worse than anyone else. Yet as each day passes it seems to get easier on him and harder on us. I still get embarrassed and upset when he loses his temper with himself for being so forgetful, which often manifests itself in violent outbursts. For the first couple of months following the diagnosis very little changed, but gradually, as his memory faded, his moods changed drastically and he became more and more depressed.

I think he has always been prone to depression (ours is a family that never speaks of personal issues, so this was never confirmed), but the Alzheimer's has magnified this to an exponential degree. There were some weekends when I would visit from London and Dad wouldn't even get out of bed. Sometimes I would get annoyed at him and shout before going down to the bottom of the garden to cry on my own because I didn't want anyone else to get upset.

It was quite isolating to start with because, as I said, ours was a family that didn't really talk much. Stiff upper lip and all that.

'What's the point of getting up?' Dad would mumble from below the safe, forgiving haven of his duvet. 'There's just no fucking point any more. I'm useless, surplus to requirements. I serve no purpose anymore. Take me outside and shoot me.'

'Well,' I would answer tentatively, 'you getting up would make everyone else feel better. Besides, none of us own a gun. You know that.'

I knew full well that this was a shit reason and would not make any difference to him. I guess what I really meant was that I wanted him to get up and carry on; to pretend that there was nothing wrong and that everything was normal. In other words, business as usual – it would certainly make my life easier. This, I know, was completely selfish, but it would be easier for everyone if things were normal again, and I so wanted this to be the case. However, I knew that with every passing second things would never be right again. Normality was a distant memory for all of us.

Today I caught Dad, as I often do, staring into space. I asked him what was wrong. I should stop asking because I know what is wrong; I don't want to labour the point by continually enquiring. I gave him his breakfast and put on the telly, but his gaze didn't alter. I cannot begin to imagine how terrifying it must be to know that you are losing your mind; to be acutely aware that in the very near future you will have to rely completely on the help of others to get through each day. Pretty soon, he may not even know.

## 30th August

I spent most of today at my friend Ellie's house trying to get a bit of a break from the family. Mum had gone shopping and Dad had apparently called her from the house phone (a very rare occurrence these days, as he doesn't always recognise it).

'Where is my passport?' he asked.

'Eh, I don't know, love, not sure – why do you want it?'

'It's my passport – I should have the right to see it whenever I want,' he snapped back.

Mum straight away recognised that Dad was having one of his 'episodes', for want of a better word.

'Are you planning on going anywhere, dear?' my mum joked.

Please note – when a person who has diminished psychological capabilities acts irrationally, joking is seldom, if ever, the correct way to defuse the situation.

Dad hung up the phone, and even though Mum tried to call him back several times, he didn't answer. Even so, she wasn't really worried – until she arrived home. Dad was back in bed. It was just after 4pm and the house had been ransacked. Random pieces of torn paper littered the dining-room table; two dining chairs were on their sides and a couple of kitchen drawers were hanging out. Mum went upstairs. The back bedroom (my old bedroom, which doubled as a study) was flooded with files and papers, tax documents, bills and books. The computer keyboard was on the floor and one of the curtains had been torn down. In the master bedroom, Mum found that all of the drawers had been pulled clean out of the chest and their contents strewn across the room. Some of the drawers had been completely snapped in half. There was a Dad-shaped lump under the duvet in the bed. It was moving slightly, shaking and sobbing. Mum pulled back the covers and, although she must have been on the verge of belting him round the ears with her handbag, put her hand ever so gently under his chin, turned his face to hers.

'I'm so sorry,' she said to him. For although in many respects Dad should have been the one to say sorry to her, I know that my mum was apologising for the thoughts going on in her head; how, since setting foot inside the house, she had come to hate this man. She felt ashamed of herself for being so mad at someone who really couldn't help it. She was also embarrassed, as her instinct had been to rip the duvet cover off the bed and scream the house down. Most of all, though, she was mortified at the realisation that things had become this bad.

Later on, Dad got up and mended the drawers that he had broken and the three of us got the place looking neat and tidy again. Dad has pretty much forgotten about it already, but Mum hasn't – no matter how hard she tries.

## 31st August

The person who is coping the worst with Dad's illness is Mum. This is no big surprise, really, when you consider that at the age of 61, my mum is still as bright as a button and has the patience of a bee with ADHD. She is very caring and kind but she is just . . . well, impatient really. I remember when she attempted to teach me how to drive; it resulted in a massive argument and we didn't speak for weeks. I am 25 now and I still don't have a licence.

Before I moved back here, Mum would call me to complain about Dad. We weren't a gossipy family or a dysfunctional one – far from it – and she wouldn't previously have had a bad word to say about anyone and certainly wouldn't have confided in me, as that would have crossed some sort of parent/teacher boundary. But I guess she had no one else to say these things to, and she would never have wanted that sort of gripe to be relayed outside of the family walls. So I became her sounding board and confidante.

'He's just so bloody forgetful,' she'd say to me. No shit. The man has Alzheimer's – he is hardly going to give you an in-depth account of everything he has done that day, is he?

Despite her closeness to her friends, Mum remains an extremely private person. To begin with, she was reluctant to tell anyone about my dad's illness. I told her that keeping it a secret was a bad idea. I was of the opinion that people needed to know, as it would surely go some way towards explaining Dad's regular, bizarre behaviour and his repetiveness. She told her friends and then eventually our relatives (on both sides of the family), and I told my friends. I also mentioned it to a couple of the local pub landlords when I was home visiting. I wanted people to know because my brother and I weren't always around. I needed to feel that there were people who understood, or at the very least were aware of our situation, and could help out if need be. It got to the stage where when I told people, they said, 'Well, we did think there was something wrong. Now you mention it, that makes complete sense.' I was glad we were telling people, and that they wouldn't just think my old man was mad.

My mum, as with most women of her generation, is a woman who has great pride; pride in her appearance, pride in her family and home, pride in what people think of her, and so on. This is especially prominent when you live in a small town like we do. Folk love to gossip, and Mum hates being the talking point of someone's coffee break. This is probably why she is so private about stuff. However, now we have started to tell people about Dad being ill, I feel pretty confident that word will get around, like it always does. Most people who come into contact with my dad will do so with the knowledge and understanding that he isn't quite all there. With mental health issues, Alzheimer's in particular, just being aware of its existence is a very important thing. So far, none of us has experienced any negative responses from people. Why would we? It's not a very nice thing to be associated with, but things could be a lot worse. Generally, people said the same thing as most of the friends who knew my dad. Something along the lines of, 'I'm really sorry to hear that, it's a real shame. I'll keep my eyes peeled for him anyway – don't you worry.'

It was nice to know that. I did genuinely feel happy that there were people looking out for him.

## 1st September

Ha! My mum and dad are going out tonight with the Alzheimer's Society. A while after my dad was diagnosed, they decided (well, obviously, Mum decided) to join the local branch. They usually do something different every couple of weeks; go out for a meal, go bowling in Newport, have someone from a local service come in to give a talk or demonstration on something. I used to joke with my mum when they had a meeting to go to by saying, 'Hey, do you think anyone will remember?' Tonight, though, has to take the prize for the best idea ever. This is brilliant . . . tonight my mum has informed me that they are having a quiz. A quiz! That's a bit rich, isn't it? Fuck's sake. Even though my mum told me that it is really for the benefit of the carers, I still pissed myself laughing. I know I shouldn't, but amusement is pretty thin on the ground these days so you have to take your kicks where you can.

## 2nd September

Mum and I decided to go to the cinema today, Dad wanted to come too. Sometimes I find myself in a bizarre quandary: either take your old man to the cinema and risk him making inappropriate comments to the fat lady in the next row, asking for sweets he doesn't like, getting lost on the way to the toilets, talking loudly through the film and getting in a fight, or leaving him alone to burn down the house. So we all went to the cinema.

Mum drove while Dad pointed out of the window at squirrels that weren't there. The cinema in town is really small, probably less than 50 seats. Back in London people go mad for small, intimate cinemas like this, perhaps the Valleys is way ahead of London for a change. Actually, don't quote me on that. The cinema is small and dingy and known affectionately by the locals as 'The Flea Pit'. There's no art deco-themed bar serving craft wines, no button to press for service, no smoked almond nuts; just chewing-gum stains on the floor and a faint smell of piss and bleach.

I remember going there for a birthday with my friends when I was really young to watch *The Land Before Time*, that cartoon thing with dinosaurs. Mum cried and I have never forgiven her for embarrassing me. Anyway, a new film has come out called *The Da Vinci Code*, and as Mum haggled with the mottled youth on the door to let her and Dad in as OAPs, the whole trip cost us less than a tenner. We strategically sandwiched Dad in between us with Mum on the aisle seat and me acting as a buffer between him and two rather amorous teens. We worried that his attention span wouldn't last the duration of the film and we agreed that if his interest waned to the point of no return that I would take him for a walk round the shops and Mum would stay and watch the remainder of the film. She deserves some alone time. But, fair play to him, he watched intently, laughed ridiculously loudly at bits that weren't that funny and seemed to enjoy himself. So two and a half quid well spent.

As we emerged back into the drab sunshine Dad took me by the hand and said, 'That was lovely, wasn't it? Good fun?'

'Yeah,' I replied. 'Did you enjoy the film, Dad?'

But he looked at me like I'd just asked him what 1245 divided by 789 was.

We went to the butcher's and got some pork chops for tea and I sat both of them down while I got on with stuff in the kitchen. We had dinner on our laps, we seem to do that more and more these days, when some chap came on the news who had alopecia. He was very pale, too, striking-looking. Between mouthfuls of pork chop, Dad pointed at the telly and remarked, 'Look, look at that man, he looks just like Silas, the albino monk. You know, from that film we watched earlier, with your man Tom Hanks!'

Mum bent over her plate laughing, cutlery clattering on the tray.

'Dad, you don't even know who Tom Hanks is!' I chortled.

'Course I bloody do, I've been watching films before you came about,' he declared proudly. '*Da Vinci* something or other, was it? Da Vinci's Book, yup, that's it, I saw that one, he looks like the fella. Oh, he's gone now. I wonder what he was selling?'

'Selling? What do you mean, Dad?'

'Oh, for God's sake love, keep up. The chap we just saw here, the chap that looked like the monk from the film, what was he selling? On *The Antiques Roadshow*,' he continued, as he jabbed his gravy-spattered knife in the direction of the telly.

We were watching the news.

### 3rd September

This is testimony to my growing belief that I should never, ever leave my parents unattended for any period of time. Last night I stayed round at my friend's house for a bit of peace and quiet. Mum has been good at ensuring I get out and see people. Plus, I think she worries I might become lazy and just want to stay at home all the time. Far from it! At around 8 o'clock, I received an odd phone call from Mum. Mums are generally worriers, it's in their nature and it's part of their job description; in short, it's what they do. I answered the phone and made some small talk, but Mum was very quiet and seemed troubled.

'Has something happened, Mum? You're very quiet. What's wrong?'

'It's your dad, love,' she said. (Would it ever be about anything else?) 'He hasn't come home this evening.'

It wasn't too late, and although we didn't like Dad to go out by himself for very long, I told her not to worry.

'I always tell him to leave a note if he is going out so that I don't worry about him,' Mum said. 'But he never does, he always forgets.'

Again, this is a common part of having Alzheimer's. There's no great surprise there.

'He's probably in the pub,' I said, knowing there were no two ways about it. That was where he was, even though we had told him on numerous occasions not to go to the pub alone any more. I told her not to worry too much and to give it another hour or so, but if she was that worried about him she should just drive into town and haul him out of his chosen drinking establishment. However, Mum was a bit funny about going into pubs on her own. She didn't really drink much – the odd glass of champagne at Christmas or birthdays, but that was it. I think she still subscribed to an old-fashioned belief that a lady oughtn't to venture into pubs without a chaperone. Unlike me.

Another couple of hours went by and I got a second phone call from Mum – he still wasn't home and she had been for a drive around town to see if he was wandering around somewhere. I told her to call the pubs and then to call me back, which she did. I went home to be with her. No one matching my dad's description or answering to his name was in any of the local watering holes. My mum then made the phone call that she really didn't want to make; she rang the local police station and was told two officers would be round to the house straight away. Now Mum was really worried, and I have to I admit so was I, so I was grateful when two of our town's finest boys in blue immediately came over. Mum just kept apologising for calling them out unnecessarily, but they kept saying that due to Dad's condition, the situation should be treated seriously. After answering a few questions and drinking several cups of tea, one of the officers stepped out into the hallway and made some calls to the local hospitals.

He came back into the room to an anxious Mum.

'OK, the hospital has confirmed they admitted a man matching your husband's description earlier this evening . . .'

Mum gasped and clamped her hands over her mouth, her sad eyes fearing the worst. I looked on, as if watching a film or something, not really wanting to believe that this was happening. It turns out that Dad was OK. A local resident had gone to put their bins out or something and found him lying in the gutter by the side of the road with a large cut on his head. They went over to see if he was alive. He was, but he wasn't making much sense. He couldn't remember where he lived, even though he was less than half a mile from the house. Neither could he remember what had happened or who to contact. He seldom took out a wallet or any form of ID. An old-fashioned guy, he just carried cash. The good Samaritan from down the road had called an ambulance and then sat with my dad until it arrived. Now, none of us could figure out who this person was, and the police didn't give their name, but I would like to thank them from the bottom of my heart for helping out where many others wouldn't. I hope that someday when they are in need, karma looks after them just like they looked after Dad.

So the police took Mum down to the local hospital – arguably the most horrible place in town – where she was let in to see a very sheepish and humble Dad, who was still very dazed and disorientated. Apparently, when the paramedics got him to the hospital he kept asking for my brother – not Mum or me. We think he had fallen in the street when he was walking up the hill, which, in his defence, is very steep. The shock, coupled with a few pints and a nasty bump, led to his delirious state. When you add this to the Alzheimer's, it's not surprising that he made very little sense. While Mum went to fetch Dad I fussed around the house, much like Mum would do, hoovering, tidying, polishing, cooking, sorting. Even though this is a complete nightmare, I'm glad I am here, for Mum more than anything.

## 4th September

I had an unusually frank conversation with my mum today. As I have said, we are not a family of openness or forthright conversation. We were in the car heading towards town to do some shopping. Dad was vague when he arrived back from hospital and I am becoming more and more aware of how hard this must be for my mum. He quietly toddled up the path to the front door, hands clasped behind his back, head down low. He gave a barely audible 'Hello, love' to me as Mum ushered him in through the front door. I made him a tea and put it on a tray with some biscuits I had made, and he said he would take them up to bed with him as he needed a rest, but they didn't make it past the dining table. Mum just crumpled down onto the sofa, coat still on and bag in hand.

It's as if she's married to a different person; her husband's mind has gone, but physically he has remained exactly the same. I sometimes think how it's a little bit like Dad has been hypnotised – he looks exactly as he did, but really the person you knew has gone. I can't remember what I said that prompted this response from my mum (in between coughing fits – she has another cold, so I am looking after both of them), but she said, 'Of course, I still love him, in a way, but that is not the person I fell in love with – that's not the man I married.'

I have never felt so sorry for anyone in my whole life. I cannot begin to imagine the isolation that Mum must be enduring. It must be like losing your husband and gaining a very needy child who just gets younger and more dependent by the day. Work is one of her outlets. Imagine that, the highlight of your day is going to work just so you can escape the draining monotony of looking after someone who is terminally ill. But while you're doing this, who looks after you? The guilt that accompanies these feelings is unparalleled. I want to write how rewarding it is to look after Dad, but it just isn't. It is sad, it is embarrassing and I don't want to do it. I know he wouldn't want this either. Don't get me wrong, I don't for a second begrudge it, and although I would love for this to not have happened, now that it has I would never think of leaving. While I would rather my situation was different, it isn't. The only thing I can do is find the strength to deal with it and make this situation the best and most comfortable it possibly can be for everyone concerned. I feel a little bit like I am directing a really shit play, where the actors keep forgetting their lines. If someone were to offer me a million pounds to leave my family now I would turn it down. I am here and I am staying. Despite all my feelings, I am proud and I am doing the right thing. I know that for the rest of my life I shall never regret it. Ever.

## 5th September

As time goes on, I am growing more and more protective of my father. In fact, fiercely so. This is something that has surprised me, as I had never believed that I would have to feel like this. Parents are there to protect their children, not the other way around. I have begun to realise that my dad is just a man – not a superhero or a god and, above all, not just my dad, but a real, average human. While I was growing up, I held the view that my parents and grown-ups in general were a force not to be reckoned with – a superior power. It has taken me the best part of two decades to realise that we are all pretty much the same. We are all just people of a different age.

I think I am becoming more protective over Dad because I doubt whether most people understand the problems he's encountering. He is at the point where he just wants to talk to anyone and everyone. When we walk down the street to get his papers in the morning, he looks at people and I can see he wants to make eye contact with them so that he can then stop for a chat. He doesn't really have much to say, but just talks random shit to strangers. It can get embarrassing. Mum gets upset because people don't realise there is something wrong with him. You can't instantly recognise that Dad has a problem because you can't see mental illness. When you couple this with the negative stigma that most of society attaches to mental illness, I can see where her problem lies, and I share her concerns.

'It's not like when you see an old man in the street who is visibly nearing the end of his life,' Mum has pointed out. 'He's probably walking with a limp or stopping every hundred yards or so to sit down and catch his breath. To the untrained eye, your father is still the picture of health.'

This is true. From a distance, my dad looks great, but when you get up close and listen to him you realise that this isn't the case. He's like a Monet painting; from afar, everything looks as it should be, but when you get near, things are all fuzzy, boundaries are blurred and you see a bewildering array of things that aren't really in order. That's my dad.

### 6th September

My sleep was disturbed by nightmares again last night. My bad dreams started when Dad's condition worsened and they have increased in frequency and in direct correlation to his ever-worrying behaviour. The most frightening thing about my dreams is that they could very well become real.

I know this is textbook anxiety – the other night I dreamed about my teeth falling out. Since I have been back here, I have dreamed about Dad more and more and London less and less. I worry that my waking hours are being directly mirrored in my sleep. I am now having dreams about him nearly every night. I see him trying to mow the lawn without watching what he is doing. I see him getting into altercations and arguments with people at the local supermarket, with me having to bring up his illness to try to get him out of trouble. I dream about him running away and the rest of us having to go out and look for him. I also dream about him in his worst possible state, unable to remember who any of us are, or who he is, or where he lives. Those are the worst dreams, because I know this is inevitably going to happen. One day (in the not too distant future) I may have to visit Dad in some sort of home; a soulless institution where people who couldn't give a shit about this once-great man are paid to wash and feed him. These are the cruellest of nights because usually when you wake from a nightmare you can console yourself that it was just a dream. This wasn't just a dream; this was the reality of seeing a parent with a terminal mental disease that eats away at his fantastic personality. This horrible illness is taking the man that used to sit me on his knee and make up the most amazing stories; the man who was strong enough to pick me and two of my friends up at the same time at my sixth birthday party; the man who taught me how to varnish the chest of drawers in my bedroom, to ride a bike, to play rugby. This was the man who was My Daddy.

## 7th September

So tonight we all sat in the living room to watch *Coronation Street*. Well, Mum was watching, Dad was vilifying her for watching, and Gareth, who was home from Plymouth for a few days, and I were maintaining impartiality.

'If you can't say anything nice, why don't you just bugger off and make me a nice cup of coffee?' Mum said to him.

A little risky, I thought, but off he marched. He was out there a while, and I counted the kettle boil at least four times. Enough time elapsed for us to almost forget about the coffee request. That was until the sliding doors opened, pushed apart by Dad's foot. He walked in beaming.

'Your wish is my command,' he said to Mum, walking towards her with his head bowed. He was carrying a tray on which he was balancing a soup bowl full of steaming hot coffee.

'Fresh from the microwave!' he proudly proclaimed and set the tray gently down on Mum's lap before producing a tea towel and a spoon.

He kissed her on the head then took his seat. Looking at the telly, he blared, 'Is this shit still fucking on?'

We said nothing as Mum ate/drank an entire soup bowl filled with microwaved coffee. As she did so, she smiled at Dad and made appropriately appreciative noises.

## *10th September*

As G was home I went back to London for the weekend – and it was great, as if I'd never left. As the train whizzed through the countryside, I felt I was getting ever closer to 'me'. I walked through to the front of the train as it neared Paddington so that I could get off close to the ticket barriers and so onto the 27 bus as quickly as was humanly possible. I loved being back in the city, seeing the buzz and excitement of tourists and Londoners alike, seeing such diversity of people, and it made me think of how everyone in Pontypool looked the same. I loved looking out of the bus window and imagining the stories of each person strolling in the sunshine of this sunny afternoon.

I saw the usual crowd and we sat in the pub in Camden just like old times, getting outrageously drunk and catching up on all the gossip concerning who had been doing what to whom. I felt as if I didn't have a care in the world. It was just what I needed:

a break, a getaway, and a bit of my old life back. I stayed at Candy and Emma's, and people came and went all night. No one slept, we just drank all night through to the next morning, then went out again. It was the best weekend I've had in a very long time. I laughed so much and though the reality of my life back home never totally evaporated, I was able to compartmentalise it and allow myself to release. I thought how I hadn't heard myself laugh in so long. When I came back I felt lighter, better and more positive. I felt as if my little jaunt away had worked its magic, and while I could easily have stayed there, away from my problems, I felt ready to come back, stronger and more equipped to cope with Dad.

But now I don't.

Mum went to the doctor's again today.

She's got cancer.

## 12th September

I can't quite get my head around what has happened. I still don't really understand and I can't find the energy or words to write. Mum has aggressive skin cancer that has formed from some apparently minor skin melanoma she had removed a year ago. I can't believe we have been so blind. When she went into hospital for something pertaining to 'women's trouble' we didn't question a thing, especially my brother, who still can't bear to hear anyone mention the word 'period'. She knew then, she knew what this was and she didn't say. So it must be really serious for her to have actually used the C word.

With echoes of when she told us about Dad's Alzheimer's she sat me down after G had left and Dad was upstairs and said that it was nothing to worry about, the doctors are doing everything they can. I noticed the absence of the classic 'they've caught it early and are very certain it can be dealt with' phrase that I always hear used when people talk about cancer on the telly. She was very calm and matter-of-fact, she didn't whimper or cry or wobble at all.

She is to have an operation almost straight away, and if that doesn't work then she is going to require chemotherapy as soon as possible. There are faint traces of the disease in her lungs, too. We haven't told Dad yet, as we don't want to upset him and we also don't know how much he will actually take in. My brother and I obviously have to make plans for Dad's care, as Mum will be too weak. G is taking this very badly, far worse than me. Perhaps I am being braver, but I suspect I am in denial. You know how the saying goes, if you can keep your head when those around you are losing theirs then you mightn't have fully grasped how fucking bad this is. I feel dizzy, like someone has smacked me really hard around the head. You know when you're little and you fall off your bike badly, for the first time? You get up and your friends are looking at you, unsure whether you're going to cry or not. You want to almost laugh it off, but your eyes are prickling with the tears that you don't want to come, their voices are far off and your vision seems blurred. I felt like I needed to steady myself even though I was sitting down, and I realised that I was not just in shock about Mum, but Dad, too. The whole fucking shitty situation.

I think my mum may be one of the bravest women in the world. Not once have I detected anything less than a Dunkirk spirit from her, even though it's clear she may not come out of this. She is busying herself by instructing her work colleagues on how to deal with any workplace eventualities in her absence, creating colour-coded manuals for every task and duty, and this seems to be taking her mind off the impending doom. In hindsight, I am kicking myself for not having taken better care of her – now I see why she has been more tired over the past few months; the cough, the bad back, the colds, the aches and pains. I just put it down to the strain of looking after Dad, but I should have seen that she wasn't as well as usual. Mum never gets ill. The worst thing is she has obviously known for a long while but didn't want to tell us, or anybody for that matter. I didn't have a clue. It has been her secret.

## 13th September

Mum has her operation tomorrow. Gareth has come home so that he can take her into hospital and I can stay at home with Dad, who still doesn't seem to really know that Mum is ill. She is carrying on as normal, but even if she hadn't been I'm not sure he'd notice. Perhaps she has thought about it so much her illness now seems trivial and mundane. Perhaps she is hiding a secret talent for being an Oscar-worthy actress. Either way, Mum really doesn't seem to be too bothered about it at all. She has assured me that it's all just procedure, and that she is under no risk from the operation and that everything will be fine. She almost has me fooled, too.

As for me, there's so much going on that it's easy to brush off weepy thoughts and get shit done. Wake Dad, give medicine, do breakfast, do washing, do ironing, do food shop, walk with Dad, ensure Dad doesn't get lost in the park, run bath for Mum, make beds, schedule hospital appointments and carers' visits.

I went to sleep last night feeling sick and when I woke up this morning something felt really weird. Something was wrong, but I couldn't put my finger on it. I was having a bit of trouble breathing and I felt nauseous. I was hot and my face was soaking wet, as was some of my hair and the pillow. It took a few seconds to realise why. I had been crying in my sleep.

## 14th September

G drove Mum to the hospital last night in time for her operation this morning and I stayed at home with Dad. We have told him that she is in hospital for a procedure. He jokingly told the man in the post office this morning that she was having a boob job. I wanted to hit him with a newspaper. I attempted to keep him busy and occupied so that he didn't ask questions, though I realised that it was really my mind I was trying to distract.

Mum was supposed to come out of the operating theatre before midday, as the surgery was scheduled for first thing in the morning. At 2pm, she still wasn't out, and by 3pm the nurses on the ward still didn't have any information on her. By 5pm my brother arrived at the hospital with Dad in the car, only to be told that Mum was in intensive care. They couldn't stop the bleeding after the operation and they were doing all that they could. I had stayed at home to field any calls and to generally hold the fort, which I realised was a stupid idea. At least if I had gone with them I could have felt like I was doing something, or if Dad was here I could have been some use to him. The house echoed and the cold seeped in as I sat alone on the sofa, facing the phone. I cried for what seemed like hours before finally dozing off. Eventually, I woke to the sound of the phone. I picked it up and heard my brother rapidly talking, but not to me.

'G? Gareth? Oi – hello?!'

'Sorry, Robs, hi, hi, it's me . . . she's OK.'

'Oh, good, that's good news,' I responded nonchalantly, as if someone had just told me that the weather would be nice at the weekend. I was still a bit sleep dazed and wondering if I had dreamed our current awful situation.

'Yeah, they stopped the bleeding. She is still asleep, but she's really out of it. I went in to see her but she was barely conscious. They've got her on a lot of morphine. She's gonna be OK, though, she's gonna be OK!' His voice was urgent and excited.

'Thank God. What are you going to do now, then? Can you see her? Are you OK? Is Dad OK? Does he know? He hasn't been inappropriate to any of the nurses has he?'

My brain had kicked into gear, so poor Gareth could hardly get a word in edgeways in my thirst for information.

'Well, I've just got to wake up Dad. He fell asleep on a chair in the corridor and has dribbled all over my jacket. Then we'll come home and all of us can come back to the hospital in the morning. You OK?'

'Yeah, yeah, I'm OK. I think I'm OK.'

They came home eventually, with piping-hot fish and chips, and we ate in silence around the table, all tired and grumpy, all in our personal, silent hell. Dad ate his fish and chips with his fingers, ignoring the cutlery I had laid out for all of us. The sharp smack of salt and vinegar was sobering and I wondered what awful shit they were feeding my mum. There was some comfort in the soggy batter and soft, warm fish. Dad ordered mushy peas which looked like sick but he seemed to enjoy them very much. Tidying away the papers and cartons I put the bag outside, lest our house stink any worse come the morning. Outside on the patio, tying up the bin bags in the cold night air and pulling my cardigan closely around myself, I looked up to the huge night sky to see so many twinkling stars and a great big moon. It was pretty and I thought it would have been quite fitting for a lovely end to a much better day. I wished upon a star, I wished upon all of them, but I know that what I wished for is never going to happen.

## 15th September

This morning we all drove to see Mum at the hospital, which is on the other side of Cardiff. Dad was in the back of the car talking gibberish and my brother and I were in the front. I felt like the parent, turning round every now and then to check he was all right in the back. I kept asking G to put some sort of child door locks on in case he decided to get out at a roundabout or traffic light or something. I don't think I'm being in the least bit over-cautious or paranoid here.

Dad didn't seem concerned about where we were going and hadn't asked since we got into the car. I wondered what he was thinking about, I wondered what he knew.

We stopped off at M&S to get Mum some nice food, as the shit they were feeding her in hospital was diabolical. I wouldn't have fed it to a rat. It always strikes me as incredibly contradictory that an institution entrusted with preserving the health of a nation would choose to feed its patients such crap. We got her some fruit, a vegetarian pasta salad, some crudites with hummus and some sparkling water. We also brought her some shortbread to keep by her bedside, though I already know she will complain about them not being authentic or Scottish enough or as good as hers. (Mental note: must look up Mum's recipe and make some proper shortbread.)

It was a very large Marks & Spencer, and as we went about our business in the food aisles, Dad wandered off into the lingerie section and I had to go and retrieve him. Twice.

Anyway, when we got to the hospital, Mum looked really well. She was sitting up in her bed, smiling and thrilled to see us. Her nightie and gown were pristine and crisp, her hair was in place and she had managed to put on a little bit of make-up. I was beginning to think (that should be, hope) that she was faking it and that there was nothing really wrong with her at all. Once we got onto her ward Dad strode majestic-ally ahead of us, taking control of the situation. He gently took her hand and kissed her head and told her that he had brought us to see her. She smiled at us wanly. We stayed by her bedside for hours, talking and reading. As well as the groceries, I had brought her magazines, puzzle books, clean nighties, underwear and some perfume and skincare samples that I had spare – a little package of love to make her hospital stay somehow more bearable.

We joked about a time when Mum had been ill about 15 years go (the only time anyone ever remembers her being unwell) and she asked us what Dad had done to entertain us that day. I said that he had taken us into town and with his pocket money G had bought a record by Houtney Whiston, as I couldn't pronounce Whitney Houston.

After the laughter subsided we realised that it was nearly dark and the time had come for us to go. The staff had prompted us several times to leave, but in a kindly way, as they knew our situation. Dad got quite upset. I think reality had dawned on him; Mum was really seriously ill and there was nothing he could do about it. He couldn't even look after himself, let alone look after his own wife. He now had to watch his children do what he felt he should be doing. He clung to her hand, a little too roughly, as she was still attached to a drip, and whimpered, 'Come back to me, my love, please come back soon.' She patted his hand like she would have done mine or G's and nodded, bottom lip wavering.

My brother and I stood by the door and let them have their time. It was an awkward and forlorn walk back to the car. To cheer ourselves up, we put on some power rock for the drive home. I love a bit of rock, I do. I reckon that should I ever be in a coma, only Whitesnake or Aerosmith or Motörhead could rouse me. If all else fails and I am beyond medical assistance, then a sharp blast of 'Here I Go Again' or 'Fool For Your Loving' will rescue me from deathly sleep and carry me back to the land of the living.

Sadly, Dad didn't agree with our choice of music. Halfway along the M4, I turned around in my seat to see if he was OK. He was squashed into the corner of the back seat, his eyes tightly shut and his hands theatrically clamped over his ears, as if his life depended on it. He was really fucked off and wanted us to know, which annoyed me. We pulled up at the house and I prodded him to let him know that his hellish journey was over.

Gareth dropped us off before having to make a hasty retreat to Plymouth, leaving me to hold the fort. I don't think it will be long until G might have to move back, too. We all hope he won't need to, but with every passing day it is looking more likely. I'd volunteered to move back in the first place so that he didn't have to; being five years further along in his career, it was a bigger sacrifice for him than me. I want to be able to handle things myself, to prove that the baby of the family has grown up, that I could manage. But now I'm not so sure I can.

I made supper for Dad and I – chicken Kievs and vegetables. Dad said that they were the best Kievs he had ever tasted and he had been to Kiev. I think that's one of the few places in the world he hasn't actually been to, but the compliment made me smile all the same. I like to feel that I had done something well. He kissed me on the head and collected our plates to take them out to the kitchen, but I caught him washing them in the downstairs bathroom.

Just before I packed Dad off to bed, he turned to me and asked, 'Darling, where's Mum? Why isn't she back from work yet? Has she gone away?'

That just blew me away. How do you tell your dad who has Alzheimer's that his beloved wife is in hospital with cancer? I took a deep breath.

'She's in hospital, Dad. We just went to see her this afternoon, remember?'

'Uh . . . oh, yeah. What's wrong with her, then?' His brow furrowing both with concern and confusion. He raised his hand to stroke his beard, the way he used to do when faced with a big puzzle at work, trying to figure out how to stem the flow of a river or redirect electrical currents.

'Cancer, Dad . . . she's got cancer.'

'Oh,' he said breezily. 'OK, will she be back tomorrow?'

*Fucking hell.*

'Uh, I doubt it, Dad,' I replied, trying to keep the frustration out of my voice.

'Well, that's a shame. I wanted to take her for a walk in the park – she likes that park and so do I!'

This was hard work. I paused and then offered an answer that wasn't so much an answer, but a response intended to defuse an awkward situation.

'Well, how about you and me go for a walk in the park tomorrow instead, then, Dad? Yeah? Just us.'

'And your brother?'

*Oh, dear God.*

'He's gone home, Dad, back to his house in Plymouth. He left about an hour ago – you said goodbye to him and then you made the wanker sign to him from the front window as he drove off.'

'Oh yeah, I do remember now, love, yeah. OK then, that settles it. Just you, me and Mum then. That'll be nice.'

'Yeah, it will, Dad. Now off to bed then.'

'All right then, darling. Oh, you're a lovely girl you are. I'm a lucky man. G'night.'

He kissed me on the cheek and rubbed my head, messing up my hair. I love it when he does this as it makes me feel like a little girl again, and him like my daddy.

## 16th September

One month home, one month away from London, and it has been the weirdest and maddest month of my life. I ruminated on this as I lay awake in bed, listening out for noises of Dad. How much is it possible for a person to change in just one month? Whenever I think of London and my life there I feel more as if I have read about it or seen it in a film. I don't feel close to it or as if I have lived it. I speak to people there as much as I can, but I guess it's hard for them to comprehend what things are like here and I don't have the time to paint that picture for them.

Dad slept in again this morning. These days, I try to let him lie in for as long as he wants, unless I have to get him up for something. As time goes on, he sleeps more and more. This gives me a bit of time on my own to eat breakfast, sort shit out and generally sit in peace and quiet until he gets up and the utter madness starts. He used to be an early riser; we all are really, no one lies in past 7.30am unless the world is ending, but come to think of it, ours sort of is!

Eventually, at about quarter to ten, Dad came into the dining room wearing just his pyjama bottoms. He was marching like a Russian soldier with his legs kicking high.

'Morning, Dad,' I said. He returned my greeting with a swift pivot turn and a salute.

'You going to get washed and dressed, then?' I asked, smiling hopefully.

'Yep,' he said, and then he wandered into the lounge and looked out of the window with his hands clasped behind his back. He sat on the sofa before getting up and going over to the window again.

'You going to get washed and dressed then, Dad?' I repeated.

'Yep, yep,' he replied, but he still made no advance towards the bathroom. After about five more minutes of gentle persuasion from me, he eventually went to take a shower. It takes him a lot longer to do even basic tasks these days, mainly because he gets distracted and forgets what he is doing about halfway through. After he came out of the shower and dressed (I put his clothes out on his bed for him most mornings, sometimes it helps him, sometimes he will spend 20 minutes rooting through his wardrobe), he came back to the kitchen and made his breakfast, which is usually a 20-minute task at least.

'Where's Mum, love? Has she gone to work already?'

'What?' I replied, in disbelief that last night's chat was stolen from his mind and replaced with a great gaping hole of knowledge.

'Where is Mum today? Is she in work?' he repeated.

'No, Dad, she's in hospital, remember?'

I really need to stop using that last word.

He dropped his spoon in shock, splashing milk and Rice Krispies onto his woollen sweater.

'Christ, love, what's wrong? What happened? Has she been in an accident?'

He panicked, his eyes wide and mouth agape. His hand went to his beard again, anxiously toying. He had totally forgotten about the previous day's activities. There was not even a hint of recollection.

'She's just had an operation, Dad. Do you remember that yesterday we went to see her at the hospital in Cardiff? The three of us?'

'Oh, yeah, yeah I do now. I remember.'

I could tell that he didn't because when he's presented with a fact he can't remember, he often just changes the subject.

'Another nice day, though, isn't it?'

'Yeah, it is, Dad. You know what, after you've finished your breakfast I think we should walk to the Tesco and get some food. What do you think?'

'Great idea, lovely girl. Oh, you look after your Dad, don't you, eh?'

But I really don't feel like I do.

## 17th September

It isn't all doom and gloom with the old Alzheimer's. Some of the stuff Dad does can be quite amusing, although in many respects I feel terribly cruel about finding humour in a fellow being's misfortune. I called my brother today, and we were talking about the time, a few months back, when I was home for a visit. I was walking back up the hill from the shops to the house when I spied Mum crossing the road. I knew it was her, even though she was quite a way off. She was wearing her vile, big, fluffy, purple mohair cardigan. I hate that bloody cardigan. It has sparkly bits in it and huge shoulder pads, and down one side it's embossed with lilac flowers. It truly is as gauche as I have described it here. I shouted out to her, with the intention of catching her up so she could help with carrying the shopping.

'Mum, Mum, wait there!' I yelled, as I struggled up the hill. 'Wait there!' But she didn't stop, she just carried on her merry way before I could get near enough to be within earshot.

I reluctantly picked up the pace and jogged up to the post office just as she disappeared around the corner. I caught up with her and was just behind her, still calling her name with exasperation when I realised, to my great horror, that it was not my mum. It was Dad. He had obviously put on Mum's cardigan instead of his own jacket or pullover, and he had absolutely no idea.

'All right, Dad?' I asked through stifled laughter.

'Well, hello there! All right, my love?' he replied, looking thrilled to see me, as if he hadn't seen me in weeks.

'What, er, what are you doing, Dad?'

'Oh, I'm out to get the lottery tickets, aren't I? And the *Western Mail.*'

'OK, so you're going into the shop then, are you? Like that?'

'Yes, yes. You coming too? Come on, I'll treat you to some sweets.'

Dad didn't give me so much as a quizzical look, but I wasn't going to miss this for the world. I was so stupefied that I followed him into the shop with a bewildered smile plastered over my face. He had teamed the cardigan – a spectacle from the Pat Butcher wardrobe of crap – with dark green cords, a plain polo shirt and a pair of hiking boots. It was hilarious.

Furthermore, it was so obviously a women's garment. Very few people in small-town South Wales experiment overtly with cross dressing, as far as I am aware.

Anyway, Dad greeted the post office staff with a bright and cheery 'good morning' and a quick hand salute (an action that he has used with increased frequency ever since). In return, they greeted him with what was perhaps an exact replica of the smile I was wearing; slightly shocked, amused, bewildered, not knowing whether to laugh or not. Perhaps they thought it was some kind of dare and they were on *Candid Camera.* They obviously thought he was a little eccentric, as they couldn't have known about his Alzheimer's. Either way, Dad got his lottery tickets and his newspapers, some milk and some sweets for me, as he had promised, and we left the shop. He was totally oblivious to the fun and amusement he had brought into the shop staff's morning. I followed him out like a little lamb, still sporting a baffled smirk. I duly trotted up the road behind him as he gleefully embraced the morning sunshine. I still cannot begin to question his choice of attire that morning. He didn't have a care in the world. This made me smile and it made me love him.

## 19th September

Mum is still in hospital, they have been monitoring her recuperation, which has been far slower than they would have liked. I actually think there is a part of her that's enjoying the time off, a bit of respite from Dad. The doctors initially said she would stay in for three days but this is the fourth and she shows no signs of being discharged just yet.

It is Dad's birthday today. One day last week we mentioned the date and Dad's ears pricked up like a spaniel with a catch in his sight. 'That's my birthday!' he exclaimed.

Damn it. We thought we could have got away with that one. So yesterday I went down to the shops and bought him a card, a box of chocolates, a copy of *Private Eye* and a Welsh Rugby key ring (there's not much choice when it comes to birthday gift shopping round here). I wrapped them up nicely before I went to bed. I was up well before him this morning and actually had to stand outside his door and ask if he was awake. When he came downstairs (in his pants), I wished him a happy birthday. This was greeted with a blank look that obviously required explanation.

'It's your birthday today, Dad, remember?'

I hated the way I had started to tag 'remember' onto the end of every statement when talking to Dad – he obviously didn't, and wasn't going to. This was my problem, not his.

'Oh, yeah, so it is. I knew that! Well, happy birthday to me it is, then.'

'Look here, Dad, there are some cards and presents for you.'

More shocked looks. I should have known that come the big day he wouldn't remember, and I could have spared myself the best part of a fiver. A fiver, yeah, I know, big spender, but I'm not particularly flush with cash since I quit my job.

'Do you know how old you are today, Dad?' I asked with trepidation, wondering what sort of answer I would get.

'I . . . am . . . 61.'

'Uh, uh . . . wrong. You are 63 today, Dad.'

He was in denial and I decided not to pursue this line of one-sided conversation. Should he choose to remain at 61 for a few more years, who was I to argue? Besides, lots of people adopt the strategy of lying about their age. It often has nothing to do with Alzheimer's.

He began to open the cards. He started with one from my aunt and uncle, then lost the thread a bit and went to look out of the window, hands clasped behind his back, still just in his pants.

'Dad, you haven't finished opening your cards yet. Are you coming back?'

He came back to the table and duly opened the rest of his cards and presents from me.

'Ooh, that's lovely. You're a lovely girl, you are. Where's Mum?'

I didn't have the heart to tell him. I was becoming increasingly aware that there were multiple situations in which it was more than acceptable to tell a lie such as, 'She'll be home later on,' knowing that he would draw his own conclusion from this and would probably refrain from asking any more questions for a while. It's the man's birthday, he ought to be allowed to think whatever he likes and I shouldn't be the one to shatter what little birthday joy he might have.

We went for a walk to get his newspapers. Him in his cords and pullover with tweed flat cap, striding out proudly, pleased to be alive; me in leggings, trainers and hoody, dawdling slightly, trying to keep up both with his pace and his positivity. We walked down the hill to the corner shop where he made idle small talk to the lady at the counter who never seemed to react with anything other than a warm smile and a laugh, her nicotine-stained fingers adorned with sovereign rings that caught on her nylon gingham tabard as she gestured around. Then we strolled through the park, taking in the leaves beginning to turn bronze, before returning to the house. I spent the rest of the morning making a chocolate cake. I felt he ought to have cake on his birthday and as Mum wasn't here to do it, I would. I wore Mum's apron, more for good luck than anything. Not that I am bad at baking – just not as experienced as she is. Plus, the hoody I had on was really expensive and even though I was wearing it to slob around the house I didn't want it wrecked.

The house felt empty without Mum. Every home needs a mum, right? It's a bit like having an orchestra without a conductor, roast dinner without gravy, going out without a handbag. I felt like I was just a pretender to her throne, trying to figure out, feebly, the optimum oven temperature for baking chocolate cake.

It was strange that now, with Mum away, I felt almost awkward about being alone with Dad. A bit like when you are round a friend's house and they have a young baby and say something like, 'I'm just popping next door for a sec . . . would you watch the baby?' You don't really want to be responsible, but you don't want to say no. Who can't look after a baby? In the same way, why should I feel awkward about spending the day with a member of my family? He was my dad, my own fucking father. When the cake was ready, I called to Dad to come and sample his birthday treat.

'Do you want a cup of tea, Dad?' He wasn't listening.

'Dad . . . Dad . . . yoo-hoo. Do you want a cup of tea? Oi?'

'All right! You don't have to shout at me! I'm not fucking deaf, you prick!'

I'm used to these outbursts so this didn't faze me much. I've learned to brush it off and assign it to the disease and not the man.

'Sorry, but you weren't listening. I made you a cake and I wanted to know if you wanted a cup of tea to go with it.'

The tone of my voice must have sounded agitated.

'Well, there's no need to shout at me. You can shove your fucking cake up your fucking arse!'

And with that he stormed off.

After a few tears and a conciliatory cigarette in the backyard, I spent a moment dwelling on whether it was actually possible to insert cake into one's rectum. I am sure stranger things have happened.

I went back into the house, convincing myself once again that it wasn't me – it was the disease, it wasn't me – it was the disease, it wasn't me – it was the disease. I had begun to use this as a mantra, an affirmation, just to keep me sane(ish). Dad was back in the kitchen looking at the cake. I felt my blood pressure rising again.

'Look, love, there's cake here – do you want a slice? I made it myself, just for us, eh? I'll make us a cup of tea, too.'

Some days you just can't win.

## 25th September

The local authorities have arranged for Dad to go to the daycare centre for an extra day a week in addition to his volunteer carer still taking him out on a Monday. This gives us more time, more support while Mum is still in the hospital. They have had to perform some sort of secondary operation as they weren't sure they got everything the first time. Not really that reassuring, is it? However, I am trying to take some sort of solace in Mum getting proper convalescence away from us, away from Dad.

It was kind of heartbreaking, though, seeing a van with other old people chug up the steep hill to our house and choke to a stop outside to load Dad on. He had been going to the day centre since before I moved home and it was something recommended by the Alzheimer's Society local care group. He would make some inappropriate joke about going on a swingers' weekend and then pull silly faces at us out of the window as they drove off. Or else he'd just flick V-signs, which always makes me laugh and not feel so awful about it. I wonder whether my guilt is purely selfish. I don't like the idea of him in a care centre. I prefer the idea of him here, with us, but he likes it there and he gets good care from people who fully understand his situation. I guess it is better for him and I ought to swallow my bitter pill of guilt and just get over it.

## 2nd October

Finally, Mum can come home today – after two weeks in hospital, they are releasing her. It has felt cold and lonely without her, and while I'm sure she's been well looked after, I worried about her every night, asleep alone in a hospital, with ill people all around her. I wanted to have her in her own home, to have us all together and to be able to pretend we were some sort of normal family with a future. My brother picked her up from the hospital while Dad and I tidied and prepared for her return. At one point he told me she had been away for a work trip and that the company expected too much of her. I agreed with him. Our excitement peaked as G's car pulled up outside the front window, and I made some last-minute adjustments to the table, straightened my skirt and wiped some butter from the corner of Dad's mouth as she walked gingerly into the lounge.

She looked rested, not like someone who had cancer – calm, happy and rosy of cheek – and although she couldn't walk very well after the operation and was very swollen in places, she did look well. Plus she was ever so relieved to be home, and that lifted her whole mood and everyone else's; it felt like a beautiful welcome home party. And it was.

The district nurses said they would be calling in every day to see her and check her progress. My brother and I took Dad out for a walk in the park so that Mum could have a bit of time on her own, though I was careful not to leave her for too long, just in case she needed something or had an accident.

I am glad to have her home, but both Mum and Dad really pissed me off this evening, bursting the bubble of domestic bliss that I had worked so hard to create. Sometimes I feel like I don't do anything right. My dad has been really difficult. He keeps doing things that constantly jeopardise everyone's safety (and my sanity). I went downstairs this afternoon to find the kitchen door shut (which it never is). When I opened it, Dad was standing there in a flurry of smoke. I could detect the overpowering smell of burned toast. Again. The vicious and sharp carcinogenic stench swirling around his hapless face.

'Hello, love! You all right? I think there's something wrong with this toaster so I'm just going to get my tools out and have a play around with it,' he said as he stalked towards it with a carving knife. I managed to wrestle it off him and avert some sort of cataclysmic explosion by saying something else needed his expert engineering attention. I never got round to what that was.

Once more, he failed to recognise that he had done anything wrong. I remained calm and merely offered to make him some more toast so that the same thing didn't recur. My offer didn't go down well and he stormed out of the kitchen, stating that he needed no help and to fuck off away from him, to let him and his wife live their lives in peace. When I went to complain to Mum (not for any reassurance or advice, merely to get shit off my chest), she shouted at me, telling me not to whinge when there were people in this world with far bigger issues than ours. I know this, but it doesn't mean I'm not hurting, and it doesn't mean that I'm OK, because I'm not OK. I am torn and I am stretched thinner than I ever thought I could be. I am tired and sad all the time. I feel alienated from the whole world, like whatever is going on outside the house is happening without the slightest concern for me. I have been forgotten about as I try to keep my parents alive.

Then when I came in tonight following a driving lesson, I discovered that Dad had thrown my portion of the dinner I had prepared for all three of us in the bin. When I made a slight (and I do mean slight) complaint to Mum that there was nothing I felt like eating in the house, she bit my head clean off. I feel alone and I feel sorry for myself, but I guess I can't possibly feel as alone as my mum does right now, or my dad for that matter.

## 4th October

G was around today, and as Dad was out with his carer, we both took Mum for her first chemotherapy appointment in the specialist cancer hospital in Cardiff. She dressed up for the occasion (isn't it mad how mums do that?) in a lovely skirt, blouse, scarf and blazer, gold earrings and matching necklace. I suppose she wanted to feel as nice as possible while they pumped her full of chemicals to rid her of her killer squatters.

It doesn't take long, the old chemo; G and I waited in the reception and that was a sad sight. Mum looks positively radiant in comparison to the others, which made me feel better; she wasn't that ill, she couldn't possibly be. Time stood still in the waiting area, people only made slight eye contact with wan smiles and sympathetic gestures, like offering tattered and faded old magazines to the person next to them. A rickety old vending machine provided the only sound, whirring and clunking into action each time someone wanted to sooth their malaise with a packet of Quavers. And the sound of the nurse's voice each time she called the name of another person who might not live to see Christmas. Or who might be spared the fate. Mum would be in that second camp, we would make sure of that.

## 6th October

At the last support meeting I was told that I would be eligible for a carers' allowance as I was looking after Mum and Dad full-time and not working, so I had no other form of income. I know it won't be much, but every little helps, according to some supermarket.

I got in contact with the local authority and they arranged a home visit to see what it was that I was doing every day. It felt a little intrusive but I didn't really mind, I guess you have to do these sorts of things to avoid people abusing the system. It's hardly like I was asking for much, but there you go. No one in our family had ever received benefits for anything so I have the dubious honour of breaking that tradition! I guess when we were young we grew up in so many odd places that benefit systems just simply didn't exist. Even when we moved here and Mum didn't work she must have thought we were all OK with Dad's money and that we didn't need any more. Plus, I think our family is incredibly proud and wouldn't want to be seen as 'spongers'.

I know I am lucky in that I don't have rent to pay, the mortgage on the house is all paid off and we have enough to cover bills and sundries, so I am in nowhere near as precarious a position as some others going through this sort of thing. Mum and Dad just think it might be better for me to have a bit of allowance of my own; laughably they said it might make me feel more independent – while depending on the state. The people at the carers' meetings said that our whole family had spent all their working lives paying taxes and contributions for this exact reason, in case some day you might need a little bit of it back, so that is what we have decided to do.

My big moment arrived when the door was knocked on by a stern-looking jobsworth with paperwork and attitude. She had the empathetic bedside manner of a Dickensian prison guard and wore a very poor-quality suit (old fashion habits, still with me). She took a seat in the living room, in Dad's seat, incidentally, right by the window. Dad walked in, looking bemused, pointed at her and said, 'Who the fuck is this?' before walking straight back out again. Bang on cue, old man.

Mum stayed with me and we went through her dry questions about what it is that I do for both of them. I ran through the routine of getting them both out of bed, administering medication, helping Mum change and dress her operation wounds, taking Dad out, making three meals and snacks every day, keeping the house right, shopping and admin. She noted everything down, nodding and humming. She told me that I was eligible for the carers' allowance, which is a stonking £46.95 a week (though not to be sniffed at really, things are really cheap around here).

'So, do I get that twice then? For Mum and Dad?' I asked the woman whose name I didn't bother to take in.

'Uh, no,' she scoffed.

'Oh, I just thought, because I'm looking after the two of them right now, until my brother moves back, so . . . so what happens in this situation?'

'Choose one,' she replied.

'What? Choose one what?'

'Choose a parent. You can only get one allowance so choose who you want it for.'

'And just ignore the other parent, do I?' I replied, the sarcasm dripping from my tone.

'That's your choice,' she countered, totally missing the point.

So I chose Dad, mainly for his brief and hilariously well-timed cameo in the afternoon's events.

## 7th October

Mum went and bought some fancy new phones for the house last month, a pair of cordless things, recommended by someone she worked with, that look like walkie-talkies from outer space. At least that's what Dad said. They're no Bang & Olufsen but they are leaps ahead of the old hold-and-dial

disc thing that we used to have by the sofa on the old
Chinese tea chest. It's sad because the old engineer in
Dad would have been impressed; he would probably
have chosen them himself after much in-depth delib-
eration, comparing prices and specifications, quiz-
zing clueless shop attendants about their capabilities
and potential before unleashing an unsuspected
lecture about the inner workings of telecommu-
nication devices across the world. Instead, when the
phones arrived Dad just stared at the box as if he had
been given an utterly foreign object. What seemed
like hours passed with him looking at the box and
smiling, then looking at us quizzically, then back to
the box, each time pushing his glasses up the bridge
of his nose, furrowing his brow and shaking his head.
Obviously, the old cogs were still turning in some
way, he knew that it was his job, his profession, to
figure this out and make it work, but once he was out
of the starting gate the path was muddled and blurry.

We managed to get them set up when Dad went
to bed; we didn't want to make him feel redundant,
but he probably already did. One of the phones is
in its little cradle in the living room and the other
in Mum and Dad's room upstairs. At the end of last
week we realised that one was missing. Because the
two are identical, I think we had just been moving
the one around the house, not knowing that its twin
had disappeared. But I have just found it, nestled
between some peas and a pack of mince in the
freezer. So that's that fucked then.

## 8th October

G has decided to move home. I told him it was absolutely unnecessary, that I could handle everything, that I could look after Dad and make sure Mum was on the mend. I know I can't and I know that I need help, his help, but I don't want to admit that and I don't want him to have to give up his life, too.

But then again, I know how hard it is and also how rewarding, in a fucked-up way. Plus, I do want him around; he always knows what to do in mad situations and is far better with Dad than either Mum or me. Dad listens to him.

Mum also tried to shake off G's offer, telling him that there really was no need, but her eyes screamed 'yes', just like mine must have done. And so, just like that, we are a family all under one roof again, except my brother is far too tall for his bed, Mum's having chemo, Dad refuses to shut the door when he uses the toilet and I have disturbing night terrors. One big, crazy happy family.

## 10th October

Not going out on a Saturday night has become somewhat de rigueur. To tell you the truth, I don't always half mind it. I have pretty much forgotten what it's like to be shit-faced and rolling around the floor of the pub with my mates listening to Guns N' Roses and smoking fags. But last night, cooking dinner for Mum and Dad was . . . eventful. I was making lasagne while Mum directed. Never a good impartial adviser, she had propped herself up against the wall of the kitchen and was peering judgementally over my shoulder, her silence screaming a thousand orders and pieces of wise advice. It didn't take long for that to change.

'Keep stirring, love . . . keep stirring the white sauce or it will go lumpy . . . It's going lumpy, stir it! Well, put some bloody elbow grease into it for crying out loud. God, let me do it.'

She pushed me out of the way and took charge at the stove. That's the problem with mothers, isn't it? They always know best.

Dad was sitting in the lounge with a crossword, filling it in with, I suspect, complete bollocks. But he looked happy enough. I told Mum several times to sit down and rest but she insisted on hobbling around the house in the hope of reducing the swelling around her wound. I could tell she was in a lot of pain, even though she tried to hide it.

I was just putting the assembled lasagne into the oven when Mum went to the toilet. Seconds later, I heard a thump and a scream coming from the bathroom.

'Mum, Mum, are you OK? Mum?' I rushed to the downstairs loo.

I heard a reply through broken sobs and pained wails.

'Oh, God, I've, eh . . . the stitches have burst and it's exploded everywhere,' she cried helplessly.

'I can't get in, Mum, you locked the door. I TOLD you not to lock this door, didn't I? Are you near the door?' In my head my voice was squeaky and terrified, like that of a scared child, but it came out calm and controlled. I had my war general head on.

'No, I'm over by the toilet. I . . . I went to sit down on it and it all split. It's popped open and it's everywhere. Please help me.'

Shit. Panic stations. What do you do at a time like this? Yes, that's right – you try to kick the bathroom door off its hinges. Like fucking Van Damme.

'Love, you'll damage the door. They cost a fortune. Be careful.'

That's the trouble with being a Scot, regardless of the seriousness of any given situation, you always think of the financial implications. I finally managed to kick the door through, breaking only the lock and cutting my trousers and grazing my shin in the process, but what I saw nearly made me sick. Even writing this now makes me queasy and disturbed. I found Mum lying on the bathroom floor at the bottom of the toilet with her pants around her ankles and her pale blue linen skirt hitched up around her waist, tie-dyed crimson red. There was blood and piss and lymph fluid everywhere. All over the toilet, all over the floor, all up the walls, the sink, the cabinet and all over my poor mummy. She was crying, having hit her head on the sink on the way down, and she was obviously in shock. Then I saw exactly why she was in shock. Where she had her skirt hitched up, both wounds were exposed. The stitches ran from either side of her stomach, down past her groin and finishing at the top of each thigh. They were wide open and all I could see was the inside of my mum. This brave, conservative lady was sprawled across the bathroom with everything on display and there was nothing she could do to preserve her modesty.

'Jesus Christ, Mum,' I exclaimed.

'Och, I'm OK really, it looks worse than it is. It's just a wee split.'

For fuck's sake, woman, I thought. You are lying in a pool of your own blood and other bodily fluids, with your innards hanging out, and you think that perhaps it looks worse than it is. I had to laugh.

'Right, eh, OK. Where is the pain worse? Is your head OK?'

'Um, yes, I just knocked it a little, but it's fine.'

'Can you see everything? Anything blurry? How many fingers am I holding up?'

I flipped Mum a V-sign. She attempted to slap my hand away.

'Right, no obvious signs of concussion, then. Shall I try to sit you up a bit?'

'Yes, please. I think we should wash all the bath-mats and towels in here, you know, love.'

'Yup. That was the first thing on my mind, too, Mum. If I could only shift your haemorrhaging carcass off the bathroom floor I could resume cleaning duties, but you just won't budge, will you?'

Humour, always use humour, when someone lies morbidly mangled on the bathroom floor. Just use humour, it's never inappropriate.

She smiled. 'I think perhaps I ought to call the district nurse.'

'Shut up a second, will you, Mum,' I said as I tried to prop her up against the side of the bath. I attempted to pull her skirt down a bit, but in the end settled for covering her with a towel.

'Right, I'm calling an ambulance, OK? We need to get you straight into a hospital as soon as we can and get you checked out and stitched up.'

'Ooh, darling – do you really think that's necessary?'

'Are you mad, Mum? Do you really think this will heal by itself? Do you think it will be fine with a plaster and some germ cream? If we don't get you to a hospital now you'll be dead by the time the lasagne is cooked. SHIT! My lasagne!'

I ran back out into the kitchen and switched off the cooker.

'Turn the heat down if the cheese is bubbling, sweetheart.'

At that moment, I couldn't have cared less if I never saw a lasagne again in my life. I wanted to throw the thing out of the fucking window.

'Yes, Mum,' I shouted through gritted teeth.

'You girls having fun in there, are you?' Dad called out.

Shit. I had forgotten about him, too. I ran back to the bathroom and stuck my head round the door.

'I turned the heat off on the dinner. Just going to see Dad.'

'Och, I'd forgotten about him,' Mum said.

I put a few more towels around her to keep her warm. I'd heard that when people go into shock they can get really cold. Then I ran to the living room.

'You all right there, Dad?'

'Me? Yeah, I'm all right, love. You girls having fun in there, are you? You sound like you are.'

'OK, yeah, we have fun, we do. You got your cup of coffee there, Dad?'

'Coffee? Oh yeah, I forgot about that, I did. Mmmm, coffee!'

'Well, OK. I just came in to get the phone. You carry on with your crossword and your coffee, eh?'

'Oh, coffee? I forgot about that. Mmmm.'

I hastily picked up the phone and ran back to the bathroom.

'You OK?' I asked, as I dialled 999.

Mum was crying. 'I'm so sorry,' she said.

I couldn't be bothered to tell her how stupid she was for even saying that.

'So you should be,' I replied instead. 'I was looking forward to that lasagne! Yes, hello, ambulance.' I waited. 'Yes, ambulance, the problem? It's my mum, yeah . . . she's just exploded in the bathroom.

No . . . I know . . . it's not funny, I'm being quite serious, actually.'

Mum was talking in one ear, as I held the phone to the other.

'Tell them I have just had an operation for lymph node cancer.'

'Yes, she has recently had an operation for lymph node cancer.'

'The stitches have burst fully on both sides.'

'Her stitches have burst fully on both sides.'

'Tell them that I am fine and that . . .'

I cut her off mid-sentence. 'God, shut up, Mum. Yeah, sorry about that, she isn't a very good patient. Yes, she is breathing and wide awake, as you can probably hear. She is lying down on the bathroom floor. I have sat her up a bit but I don't really want to move her too much. I've tried to stop the bleeding with towels. I think it has pretty much stopped but the wounds are gaping wide and there's all kinds of gross stuff everywhere . . .'

'Lymph node fluid,' squeaked Mum.

'Sorry, lymph node fluid,' I retold the operator, dry retching as I spoke. 'OK . . . OK . . . yes, I'll open the door so that they can come straight in and I'll sit with her . . . thanks . . . thank you so much, but please hurry.'

I hung up the phone. 'They're sending a limo for you now, OK?'

I crouched down at her side and touched her hair. She was still in tears.

'I only wanted to have a pee,' she whimpered.

Although this was quite funny, I also started to cry, before pulling myself back together again. 'Right, no time for this, let's try to stand you up!'

I took charge again. It didn't go too well. Mum stumbled and nearly fell again, crying out in pain. I set her back down on the floor.

'Go and get me a bag,' Mum said. 'Just in case I have to stay in.'

'Righto,' I said. 'What do you want?'

Mum reeled off a load of things and I raced out to get an overnight bag and pack them. On the way I ran in to check on Dad again.

'You all right in here, Dad?'

'Oh, hello, love – I had forgotten you're visiting us. Are you girls having fun out there? Sounds like you are!'

'Ooh, you know us, Dad!'

'Ha ha, yes. Ooh, you're a lovely girl, you are, eh?'

'You all right there with your coffee and crossword?'

'Coffee? Oh yeah, I forgot about that. Mmmm coffee.'

I made a swift exit and went about getting Mum's stuff together. First, I opened the front door and switched on the front yard light, so that the ambulance could find us. I felt like I was on *The Crystal Maze,* the game show with that bald bloke. I was running around trying to do everything within 60 seconds. I miss that programme.

I ran upstairs to Mum and Dad's room and grabbed a flight bag. I put in it several pairs of knickers, some nighties, Mum's entire plethora of medication, some T-shirts, some make-up and her wash bag. I then flew back down to the bathroom, taking the stairs two at a time.

Mum had positioned herself upright against the side of the bath and was making an attempt to wipe the blood and muck off the floor. Like a scene from a horror movie it seeped everywhere, its thick crimson swirls engulfing my lovely mum.

'OK, here's your bag with everything in it.'

'Thanks, love. What shall we tell Dad?'

'Leave it to me.'

I ran back through to Dad, just as he was getting up. 'What you up to, Dad?'

'Hello, love, I'm off to find some coffee. Do you want me to get you some, too?'

'Dad, there's a cup of coffee by the side of your chair. Look.' I was trying not to lose my patience.

'Oh, my coffee! I forgot about that.'

Dad slapped his hand on his forehead and giggled. 'Oh, you know, love, my brain is not what it used to be!'

'Listen, Dad. Mum and me are going to go out for a bit. We just have to go and pick up some medicine from the chemist, OK? We won't be gone too long and when we come back we'll have some dinner.'

'Oh, lovely girl, don't you worry about me, love, you know what I always say – never let the bastards grind you down. He he he . . . Well, I can always look after myself and you know . . .'

'Hang on, Dad. I'll be back in a minute. Sit down and finish your coffee.'

I ran back to the bathroom. 'Right, they should be here in a minute. You ready to go?'

'Yes. Have you called your brother?'

G was away visiting friends, getting some respite. Why did stuff like this never happen on his watch?

'No, I don't want to worry him just yet. I'll wait to see what they say at the hospital. I've switched the oven off, I've told Dad that we are just going to get some medicine, I've opened the door for the ambulance and I have your keys. What else do you need?'

Mum looked down at the floor and her face started to crumple with the imminent flood of tears, staunch parental barricades only just holding back the deluge.

'Thank you. I'm glad it's you here and not anyone else.'

She welled up again and I started to cry. Everything suddenly seemed still and quiet, a moment of calm amid the storm. And she took that moment to just be Mum, not a victim, not a cancer sufferer. She stroked my hair and kissed my hand that was resting on her shoulder and told me I was a good girl.

Then the moment broke sharply.

'Hello. Anyone in here? Hello! Paramedics here!' Thick, gruff Welsh voices rippled through from the front door.

'OK, Mum, I'll get them in here,' I said, gently unwrapping myself from her.

By the time I got through to the dining room, two ambulance men had come in and Dad was up to greet them.

'All right, boys? Can I get you a drink or anything? Beer? Whisky? I'm doing the crossword, I am.'

Honestly, it takes him half an hour to make a cup of coffee, but whenever he isn't needed he's up like a shot.

'All right, Dad,' I interrupted. 'These men are here to give us a lift to the doctor's, they are. To get Mum's medicine like I said, yeah?'

'OK, tea? Coffee? Something stronger for you boys?'

The men looked a bit bemused. 'Um, no thanks, sir, we're all right.'

I quickly took charge of the situation. Dad always throws me with his bizarre behaviour and it sometimes takes a moment to get back on track.

'Sorry, she's in the bathroom. It's back there, beyond the kitchen.'

I turned back to Dad and placed my hands on his shoulders. 'Now, Dad, can you do me a favour for a second and . . . um . . . have a look at what time the rugby is on tonight?'

I hoped putting him in charge of something would distract him enough to let the ambulance men do their job. I needed to get Mum out of the house without Dad seeing her, as I knew it would scare the shit out of him.

'OK, love. Will do.'

He sat down with the TV guide and the remote control, squinting at the telly and pushing his glasses further up his nose. I ran back to the bathroom, where the two ambulance men were helping Mum to her feet. I gave her a bathrobe from the back of the bathroom door and she placed it over her shoulders, as if it were a prize mink fur shrug and she was about to be escorted onto the red carpet.

Mum had one paramedic on either arm as they led her through the house.

'Right then, my lovely, let's get you out of here, then. Your carriage awaits.'

Still desperate not to let Dad see her like this, I nipped ahead of them and through into the lounge, drawing the sliding doors quickly behind me. Dad had clearly forgotten my challenge about finding out what time the rugby was on, and he was sitting reading a book while the TV blared in the background.

'Dad, we're off. We won't be long, OK? We can have dinner when I get back, but make sure you eat something if you get a bit peckish, OK? There is a lasagne in the oven.'

No response.

I quickly looked around the house to see if there was anything I had forgotten, then I sped back to the bathroom and stuffed all the towels and mats into the washing machine, putting them on a hot wash. (It's becoming evident that I am turning into my mother. In a time of crisis, only a fool would forget to put a load on.)

Hurrying to get to the ambulance out front, I checked on Dad one last time.

'Dad, I'm off now, I'll see you later. Don't go out, just do your crossword and drink your coffee, OK?'

I was halfway out of the door when I swear I heard him say, 'Oh, yeah . . . coffee . . . I forgot about that. Mmmm.'

I climbed into the back of the ambulance, where the second paramedic was talking to my mum. It was then I took my first proper breath in about half an hour.

'So, are you feeling OK? Shaky? Dizzy?' he asked.

'A bit,' I replied. 'But I think it's because I haven't had my tea.'

'Um, actually, I was talking to your mother!'

Mum laughed and so did I, but only because if I hadn't I would have cried and not stopped.

'OK, then,' the paramedic continued. 'I just want to take some contact details if that's OK? Phone number?'

'What? Mine or my mum's?' I asked, not really thinking.

The paramedic behind the wheel started to laugh. 'Give it a bloody rest, will you, Geraint? I know it's a Saturday night and all, but stop chatting up the girls!'

'Hey, Rhys, she offered!' Geraint replied.

My mum was laughing, too. 'Do you think we can concentrate here, fellas?'

'Been busy tonight, have you, driver?' I called out to Rhys.

He laughed.

'Yeah, you know, the usual. Pissheads in Ponty having a fight and all that kind of thing.'

'Which way are we going?' my mum asked. 'Because I think you just took a left out of the turning when it's actually quicker if you take a right to the bottom of the hill and then through town.'

'Mum, give them a break, will you!'

'Sorry, love.'

'So, have you had a nice night then?' Geraint asked me.

'Oh yeah, just great,' I replied.

'Well, it's just as exciting as your typical Saturday night out in London, isn't it?' Mum cut in.

'Mum, an exciting night out in London is seeing Kate Moss pass out at a gig, not your mother explode in a bathroom.'

We pulled into the hospital and Mum was rushed away for assessment. I was told to stay put and wait until further news. By this time Geraint and Rhys were long gone and I never got the chance to thank them.

I decided to go outside and have a cigarette. I lit one, sat down on the concrete and then cried my eyes out. I don't know why really, I felt a bit stupid for crying, I kept thinking, 'it could be worse', and I knew it could. After all, it wasn't me that was ill – if anyone should be crying it should be my mum, but she had managed to keep it together.

When I got back to the bay where Mum was, the doctor said they were transferring her to a ward on the seventh floor and that she would be staying in for a while. I went up with her and waited around, as more doctors poked and prodded her, as if she was a piece of meat. I don't know how she put up with that. They had all the information about her cancer, or the 'stuff', as she referred to it, still not bringing herself to utter the C word at any level more than a barely audible whisper.

After about three hours or so, Mum made me go home. I was in half a mind to try to stay the night with her and call my brother to go and look after Dad. But Mum insisted that she was fine and that the hospital staff were overreacting, and I thought it was kinder to G to let the night's events wait until the morning. They will try to stitch her up properly on Monday, when the doctor who performed her initial operation is present. Until then, they'll keep her under observation and treat the wounds.

'Are you going to be all right?' I asked her.

'Of course,' she replied, as if there was nothing wrong at all. 'I feel better already. Go home, get that lasagne out of the oven and feed your father.'

'OK, I'll come back first thing in the morning.'

'Thanks, darling.'

She grabbed my hand and pulled me close. 'I love you,' she said.

This is the first time I have ever heard her sound frail and old, and it scared the shit out of me. I think I must have been looking at her the way she used to look at me when I'd fall off my bike as a child and really hurt myself. Or the time I had to have a tooth taken out under general anaesthetic and came round crying for my mummy. Our roles have switched. Everything has changed.

'I love you too, Mum.'

I held it together until I reached the taxi rank outside. Then I cried all the way home. I managed to stop for a moment to call Dad.

'Hiya, Dad! It's just me. You OK?'

'Hello, lovely girl.'

'I'm just on my way home now. I shouldn't be too long, OK?'

'Oh, you're always welcome here, love, you know that. It'll be nice to see you. I tell you what, I'll put the kettle on and you can tell me all about life in the big smoke, eh?'

He didn't even remember that I had been there just hours before. He didn't remember the ambulance, the paramedics, that Mum wasn't there, that there was a foul stench of burned lasagne and bodily fluids engulfing the house. Nothing. That shit is etched in my brain and on my eyes. He, however, was blissfully unaware of the chaos that had erupted that evening.

By the time I got home he had forgotten that I had even called and had gone to bed. I stood outside his bedroom door, checking he was asleep and listening to him snore. Then I went downstairs and ate cold, burned lasagne in the dark on my own.

## *12th October*

It turns out that things with my mum are not OK; they are very fucking not OK. In fact, things are far worse than we had expected. She has an infection in her wounds, and this has got progressively worse, meaning a longer stay in hospital. Gareth and I have spent the last few days cleaning the house, making Dad three meals a day, walking down the hill to Tesco and then walking back up again with the shopping, unless G has driven. I've ensured Dad has taken his medicine twice a day and taken him to see Mum during the visiting hours in the afternoon, staying for as long as we can each time, reading newspapers and doing quizzes. Mum is good at the quizzes but Dad obviously isn't up to his usual standard. Today I decided to take some of the question cards from Trivial Pursuit, with hilarious consequences. In the split second it takes him to turn the card over from question to answer, Dad forgets the colour code he is looking for. Apparently, the longest river in the southern hemisphere is Fatima Whitbread. Who knew? Other amusing revelations include that Marianne Faithfull founded psychoanalysis and that Portugal is the capital of South Korea.

Most of the time G is here with his car, but when he isn't we struggle to get about. Sometimes Mum's friends or our neighbours give us lifts, other times we take the bus. Dad likes the bus journeys the most.

He always remarks on what a good service the local council run. Mind you, he has a free OAP bus pass, so I suspect that travelling without any time restrictions or having to cough up for a fare constitutes a very good bus service indeed. He always tries to talk to people, and although most folk in small towns do chat on public transport, I find it draining, probably from years of travelling the London Underground in stony silence, focusing only on the patch of floor right in front of my feet. I have to keep a close eye on Dad, as you never know what might come out of his mouth next. Sometimes he's sweet and friendly and at other times he's downright inappropriate. It's occasionally apparent that the other person just doesn't want to be involved with the conversation – apparent to everyone but Dad, that is. I always try to seat him by the window. This allows me to defuse a potentially awkward situation with greater ease. I can keep him talking to me and hold his attention by pointing at things out of the window – the houses being built by the old common grounds which he loudly lambasts for being ugly or crudely proportioned – and I know full well that there must be someone overhearing this who lives in them. He embarrasses me sometimes, and I feel guilty and disgusted with myself for that. He is my flesh and blood – my daddy – and he is ill.

I think Dad is getting tired of me, too. We've had a few more rows and, unfortunately, I have lost my temper with him. He has always been a moody old grudge-bearer, but these days his reaction to certain situations can greatly vary. He will either forget that he has just told me to fuck off, or he will apologise for being ill and say that he wishes he wasn't this way. That's when I feel most sad for him. I should be so much more patient with him, but sometimes after you've woken someone up, made them three meals a day, administered their medication, made sure they've washed and changed, taken them out for a walk and listened to the same story eight times before putting them to bed, only to be scowled at and told to stop interfering, it's about all you can do to keep your mouth shut and not yell, 'Go fuck yourself!'

As I write this, I'm crying with horrid anger at myself because I should never think these things. I feel sick when I think about how angry I've been at him. I love him so much and I only want to help him. If I knew that anyone else thought of him like this I would be furious. If someone tuts at him for standing in their way at the supermarket, I stare them right in the face, with my hand on my hip and my head on a tilt, and say, 'I'm sorry, can I help you with something?' How dare anyone hold anger towards someone who is unable to control their actions?

I'm hoping that this time at home caring for Mum and Dad is making me a stronger and more tolerant person. When you spend a few days with totally incapable adults, it makes you see things differently. Life becomes more basic. I am aware that I am changing. I have often been that angry, rushed person in the supermarket, tutting at people who were in my way and never stopping to think there may be a reason for their stillness or confused expression. I'm not saying that I don't miss my old life, but there are certain aspects of it that seem so unimportant now. I'm not reading *Vogue* so much and feel somewhat indifferent to the fickle world of fashion. But I miss my friends and not having any responsibilities. I miss going to gigs every night. I miss long evenings in the pub talking random shit to random people. I miss those long Saturday afternoons on Primrose Hill that morphed into Saturday night and Sunday morning.

However, this pales into insignificance when you have just spent the previous week helping your mother change her underwear and watching your father slowly lose his mind.

## 17th October

I went to see Mum on my own today. I'd taken Dad for an early walk in the park, fed him his breakfast and medication, settled him down with a newspaper and the telly and told him to stay put. I decided to call a taxi, as it was quicker and I was cautious about leaving him alone for any longer than was absolutely necessary. I suppose I should have just taken him with me. I ought to have known better.

I took Mum some flowers, fruit and newspapers and we sat and talked about nothing for an hour. She seemed tired and said she wasn't getting much sleep because there were people coughing and stuff, but I think it's because she's in a lot of pain. I'm no doctor but I sneaked a look at her medical chart at the foot of her bed and that's a shit load of drugs she's on. We consciously avoided talking about Dad, as I knew it would stress her out. Also, it was implied in my silence that all was well.

After about an hour and a half, I said, 'Well, I guess I ought to think about getting back, I don't want to leave him for too long on his own.'

'No, you're right, love,' Mum replied. 'It was wonderful to see you and I think you've lost weight again.' Always a bonus, I thought.

As I stood up to leave, I thought I could see Dad walking across the ward.

'There you are, my love!' he called, striding towards us with a bunch of flowers and what looked like a quarter of sweets in a brown paper bag.

I looked at Mum, who, like me, was utterly astonished. We both just stood there, our mouths hung wide open, eyes narrowed.

He leant over and kissed her head. 'I've gone and got you some flowers and bought you some cough sweets for your cold. I'm sure they'll make you all better.'

Then he took her hand and let out a big sigh.

'Hey, Dad,' I began. I looked at Mum, who still

had her mouth wide open. 'So, eh, how'd you get here this morning?'

'Well, I got the bus here, didn't I? Had to change once but that's fine with the old pensioner's bus pass.' He tapped his chest pocket and smiled knowingly, as if he was getting one over on the system. 'I just wanted to get here and see how my girl is.'

He took Mum's hand again. And that was that, pretty much.

We didn't choose to probe Dad on his mysterious appearance. He might not have given any rational answers anyway. In a sudden clearing from the haze of dementia, he must have risen from the sofa, understood his wife was ill, remembered what hospital we must have told him she was in, picked up some cash and his bus pass and made his way to her – a bit like a homing pigeon or a really loyal dog. The flowers were pretty, the cough sweets were revolting and the sentiment was unquenchably dear. I let my parents chat while I went to the loo, spoke to some nurses and tidied the things in Mum's bedside cabinet. When the nurses started to hover, I made moves to get Dad back into his coat and tweed flat cap. He didn't want to leave. He got tearful and said he would never leave Mum's side. He grasped at her hand and squeezed her arm, which I'm sure must have been sore, her veins battered and bruised from countless blood tests. He kept saying he would take her home and perhaps they could go on holiday to cheer her up. I eventually managed to get him away, briefly kissed a still very puzzled Mum and said I would call in again tomorrow.

I still have no idea how Dad managed to get to the hospital today. It's not an easy journey and the walk from the bus station takes about 20 minutes. I'm not sure I could have directed him to the hospital even when he was in a good frame of mind, let alone now. He was obviously lucid and aware during the journey, but that time was now up. The radio that was his brain was tuning out again, signals fading, coherent sounds growing dim, the senseless crackle taking over.

I got him back onto the bus and let him sail to his seat after flashing his OAP bus pass, while I rattled around for some change.

'Where we off to now then, love? Another adventure? Will we catch a train this time? Scotland? A holiday?'

And with that, I realised Dad was mad again.

### 29th October

Yesterday was my birthday. I completely forgot. I am now 26 years old.

### 31st October

My brother and I went to see Mum in hospital today, leaving Dad with his merry band of dementia friends for the day. Mum seemed brighter and more positive, she was smiling and had managed again to put on a little bit of make-up. Then her doctor came and sat with us. She looked mournful and evasive. Her news? Mum's tumours have spread far and wide: to her lungs, kidneys and lymph nodes. The little fuckers are everywhere and there is nothing we can do. There's nothing anyone can do. Mum looked at us for help, the only time I think I have seen real panic in another person's eyes, the fear of knowing that your days are numbered, your time is up. G and I sat mute, each holding one of her hands, waiting for the doctor to change her prognosis, to say she got it wrong, to apologise – she had been looking at someone else's information, anything, just be wrong on this. Say she's better, say you can help her. Tell us you can save her.

Mum wants to come home.

## 2nd November

We brought Mum home today. Gareth went to collect her from the hospital. I stayed at home to ensure everything was clean and tidy. Dad was excited about Mum's return. He put on his best shirt and gave his beard a trim. We also went to the market and Dad picked out some flowers – faintly scented pink lilies, just bursting open with long, velvety petals stretching out to greet the world. Dad knows these are her favourite. He told the florist that they were for his wife, who had a very bad cold and a tummy bug. He said that when they first got together, he had taken a bunch to her flat in Chelsea. I don't know if it is a true story but it is a nice one.

The sun was shining as we walked back up the big, long hill to our house, and I linked my arm through Dad's. We opened the back doors and windows and let the sweet smell of the garden's last remaining jasmine waft through the dining room. I changed the table linen and laid out some tea, coffee and some of the cakes and biscuits I'd made. I was trying my best to emulate Mum's culinary excellence, and I was failing miserably. They tasted OK, but they looked like shit.

Mum seemed so excited to be home, as if it were a new beginning, a fresh start, like when you move into a new house. She couldn't stop touching the table linen and smelling the flowers. Dad was thrilled to 'have his girl back', too, though he did ask her how her cruise with her friends had been. I don't think anyone in our family has ever been on a cruise, or even expressed any desire to go on one. Nevertheless, she smiled and told him the cruise had been lovely.

We ate cake and drank tea, except for G who has always had a distinct dislike for hot drinks. The only time I have ever seen him drink tea was when he got knocked off his old bike when we were kids; a neighbour recommended it for the shock or something. So today he had some fizzy pop instead. We had never been allowed fizzy drinks when we were kids, except on holiday or on special occasions. But this afternoon, sitting round the table all laid out like it was someone's birthday, seemed like a special occasion. And it was in a way, it was a lead-up to a goodbye.

Mum was wobbly on her feet when we helped her up to bed some hours later. We'd made her room up all nice, filling it with more flowers, books and magazines. We'd put a jug of water by the bed with slices of lemon in it and placed next to it a cowbell, which she could ring for attention. It was the nearest thing we could muster to an intercom. Dad was relegated to the spare bedroom (my brother's room), while Gareth had the box room with the tiny single bed in it (my room). How he is ever going to get a good night's sleep in that I'll never know, the goon is nearly 6 foot 3. Meanwhile, I got the sofa in the living room, piled with cushions and old tartan blankets that smelled of our long drives in the car to Scotland. Clutching them closely I tried to slumber and think of our happy childhood, but everything was now inescapably different.

## 5th November

Aunty Judith, Mum's younger sister, has flown all the way from Scotland to stay with us. The story goes that when I was really young I found Judith far too complex a name to pronounce, so I called her Aunty Juicy instead. So, Aunty Juicy is staying in the box room and G is going to be sleeping in the living room with me. Mum and her are very close and Judith wanted to be with her, with us, to help us. I didn't want her to help me, I wanted her to be able to spend time with Mum so they could read, talk and do whatever they wanted. My aunt was shocked to see how much Dad has deteriorated. I guess we don't notice it because we see him every day. But she was more shocked to see how much Mum's health has gone into decline. Then again, we can all see that: she has lost weight and her colouring seems off, like when your favourite sweater is faded after too many washes.

Any fears I had of an outsider disrupting our family unit dissolved as soon as Aunty Juicy arrived. She's been warm and kind (as always) and has really helped lighten our load. She's helped with the washing, cooking and cleaning, and she's assisted us with Dad. Plus, I think she looks like our mum, she acts like her and sounds like her, too; it's like having more Mum! Most of all, she's helped boost Mum's mood. I think Dad likes having her around, too. He keeps saying it's like the good old days and how nice it is to have all the family back together again, even though only part of the family are together and it's nothing like the good old days.

Last night, we were sitting round Mum's bedside chatting and reminiscing, when Dad said, rather philosophically, 'You know what? We've been so lucky, as a family. We have travelled the world, we have two wonderful children, we have a lovely home and we have shared some wonderful experiences.'

We all nodded, smiling softly.

'And, we've never really had a day's illness in our lives!'

Dad was totally serious. I thought Judith was going to slap him. I had to leave the room, as I didn't know whether to laugh or cry. My brother went for the first option. I could hear him and Mum laughing as I went down the stairs and Dad saying, 'What? What?'

This morning, Dad thought it was Christmas. When he came down from the bedroom, the rest of us were up already; my mum, aunt, brother and I were sitting around the dining-room table drinking tea and eating toast. Dad burst into the room shouting 'Ho ho ho!' with a Santa hat on. Fuck knows where he'd found that. We all just stared at him, open-mouthed. He stood all of us up in turn and kissed us and wished us a Merry Christmas. He then went to the bathroom and by the time he came back out again (without his top on), he had forgotten that he had thought it was Christmas. Inside I really felt like I was laughing, but the laugh never came out.

I took Dad out for a walk while my brother took my mum and Judith for a drive. The air was sharp and I had to tuck my nose inside my scarf; it was one of Mum's old floral ones and smelled of her perfume. Dad had come downstairs ready to leave in a T-shirt, so I had to take him back up to their room and help him pick out a shirt and pullover and then put him in his wax jacket, scarf, gloves and flat cap. As we strolled through the park, he kicked up crunchy leaves so that they rained back down on us. He told me how he used to love walking me through this park when I was a baby, though this couldn't be true as we didn't live here until I was five. Down at the bottom of the park we could see some people getting ready to make a bonfire, piling wood into a pyramid and stuffing the structure with paper and twigs. Dad wanted to go and help but I had to distract him. We walked round the rugby pitch and he gave a good speech about his beloved Pontypool rugby club, the Welsh front row, the good times he'd had at the club. Those good times inevitably involved Mum waiting outside in the car until the landlord decided he'd well and truly had enough of him and demanded he go home! It was a beautiful ground, and as he stood with gloved hands grasping the railings I wondered what would come out of his mouth next. But as we set off on another lap of the pitch, Dad seemed lucid.

'You know, love. We've had a good innings, me and your mum. We've done lots of things, raised two wonderful children, seen the world and been blessed in so many ways . . .'

It was very similar to what he'd said the previous night. Steam formed from our mouths as we breathed in the dusk.

He tailed off, stopped walking and the tone of his voice changed. 'Will I still live here if she dies?'

I stopped and turned to face him, taking both of his hands in mine. The gloves made it cumbersome, and I grappled for close contact of fingers underneath the heavy fabric.

'God, Dad, of course! We'd never leave you, of course you know that!'

I put my arms round his shoulders and wanted to hug him all up. Is this what it feels like to have a child? To be a parent? To worry so much for someone who depends upon you, to hold their feelings of safety so far above your own?

I felt heartbroken that he had even been considering this, even if it was for only a moment.

'We'll stick together, we're family. It wouldn't be any other way. Don't think that!'

How awful to have a moment of realisation that you may lose your wife, your home, your family and your mind.

## 11th November

Mum didn't get out of bed today. This is the first day since she fell ill that she hasn't managed to get up, get dressed, put on her make-up and make her own way downstairs, as if nothing was wrong. She is too weak. I made her some porridge, even though the smell and sight of it makes me feel sick. I took it up to her room on a small tray and fed her with the spoon, as if she was a baby. She doesn't deserve to be like this. It's as if her grace and elegance have been stolen from her while she's been sleeping, by some selfish thief who won't even use them.

After the porridge, I tried to give her some medicine, but she refused to take most of it. I think she has given up.

She slept for a while, then my aunt sat with her and read aloud some articles from *Woman & Home* magazine. I don't know if Mum could hear her or not, but I like to think she was listening. I don't remember if I paid attention while Mum read to me as I slept as a child, but it's comforting to imagine that her words were absorbed somehow, even if it is only the notion that someone is with you and that they love you deeply.

I took Dad out for a walk around the park again. The good thing about having a limited memory is that you can never get bored of walking the same route around the same park every other day. I don't know if my dad would have got bored if he hadn't been ill – I suspect not, as he really loves that park.

'What time is Mum home from work today?' he asked.

I rarely flinch at these obscure questions now. 'She's at home, Dad, remember? She's ill in bed.'

'Oh yeah, Christ, yeah. So when is she going to get better then? These stomach bugs can be nasty, can't they?'

'Yep, you're right, they can be real nasty. We're not sure, though it's pretty serious . . . um . . . I suppose we should really prepare ourselves for the worst, you know.'

I wasn't sure how much of this was going in. We had sought advice from the Alzheimer's group about dealing with this situation and they advised that honesty was always the best policy, but to be led by Dad's reaction. If he didn't seem to be too upset then we oughtn't to labour the point by reiterating how monstrous this whole situation was. In order to try to retain a semblance of professionalism, I imagined that this wasn't happening to us, that I was talking about someone else, to someone else.

I continued. 'But you should always remember that you have me and that we will all be OK together.'

'Well, I'm so lucky that I have my children. You're a lovely girl, you are. Oh, you look after your old man, eh?' he responded with unnerving cheer and optimism. 'And Mum and me, well, we've had our innings and we've had a very nice life and done lots of things and . . .'

I stopped listening: it was the same speech that I had heard a million times before. He clearly doesn't quite grasp the full seriousness of the situation. I know this is probably a blessing, though. If he hadn't been ill, I doubt whether we could even begin to console him.

We arrived home. Doctors and nurses came and went. Dad thought they were for him and did the old routine of making jokes about nurses coming to visit, with the odd sexual innuendo thrown in for good measure. I could bloody throttle him sometimes. My brother and I spoke to the doctor as we showed him out of the house.

'How is she looking then . . . honestly?'

'Honestly, it's not good. She's not got long now. Um, I guess if there is anyone else whom she should see then . . . then just get them here now, there's not much time left. Any other family, close friends, anyone she might want to see to say . . . you know.'

He looked down to his hands and fiddled with a pen. Although this was stuff we knew, it was stuff we didn't want to hear. Up until that point I had still harboured the tiniest hope that he would say she was looking better, that maybe, maybe she might be OK after all. But this hope was now fully extinguished. Both G and I stood like sentries, solemn and straight, taking the blows.

'And your dad, well,' he continued, 'I'm not sure how best you ought to tackle that because these things can have a huge and profound effect on dementia sufferers, and you ought to know that he might not recover from the loss, either. Sorry. You have my number and the numbers of the district nurses. We are here for you. I've got to go now.'

And with that he walked hurriedly down the street and got into his car. When he drove past I am sure I saw our GP, the consummate professional, dabbing at his eyes at the wheel of his car.

We slumped into the walls of the narrow hallway, looking at each other and not needing to talk. To cry was not enough, to complain was futile, and there were no tears or complaints that would even come close to the mire of shit we were buried under.

So, with that, we started to make all the necessary phone calls. Aunts, uncles, best friends and old friends have been summoned to Mum's bedside. I suspect I shall have to go and get more tea bags. And gin.

## 18th November

My other aunts and uncles arrived from Scotland today. We held court in the lounge and, one by one, or two by two, they went up to sit with Mum, taking books, stories and music, and some snacks or drinks. Her cousin from London also came to visit with his wife. People stayed for hours, as Mum wasn't always conscious for long enough to have proper conversations with everyone. She still knew exactly what was going on, though. At one point today, I was sitting on the bed with her while she slept. My aunt – her sister – and her husband were standing by her bedside. My uncle had taken a boiled sweet from the bag that one of Mum's friends had left for her. All the treatment and medication has left her with an extremely dry mouth, so aside from using the artificial saliva in a can that the doctor has prescribed (yes, you read that correctly – fake spit in a tin), the sweets are the best option. No sooner had my uncle unwrapped one of the boiled sweets and popped it into his mouth, Mum woke up from her supposed deep slumber and snapped, 'Tell your husband to stop nicking my bloody sweets!' We all snapped our necks round to look at Mum, who still appeared to be fast asleep. By this time, my uncle had already coughed the offending confectionery into the palm of his hand and backed out of the room swiftly. The old bat doesn't miss a trick, I can tell you.

Dad seemed to enjoy having people round today. I know he doesn't really understand what's going on. I think he believes these people are all there to see him. He got out his old photos and maps of Africa and China and told people stories of the things he has done, the memory blanks filled in with generous fibs. Every once in a while, we had to remind him why everyone was there. Then we would take him upstairs to see Mum and each time we did he would remark on how much better she looked, even though she didn't. He kept saying, 'Look at her eyes sparkle, like when I met her, such beautiful eyes, still got that sparkle!' He would sit and talk to her for a bit and then kiss her hand and tell her how much he loved her. At those moments, I think he knew deep down exactly what was going on, but in a flash – in a single moment – that was gone and he was my mad dad again.

## 24th November

Today was much the same as yesterday. Some of Mum's friends came to visit. Each time she falls asleep now, she is unconscious for longer. We have been told to expect this and that is why we are getting people here now, as soon she will fall asleep for ever. I made tea, Dad made jokes, my brother played chaperone and friends left with tear-stained faces.

Mum's two best friends from London came to visit. They had been her bridesmaids and only around two months ago had come to take her out for lunch. They were obviously shattered to see her decline. Their best friend and companion through the journey of their younger years was now lying barely conscious and close to death. I left them with Mum to say their goodbyes and, as I crept quietly down the stairs, I heard one of them ask her to get the gin and tonics ready 'on the other side'. When they eventually came back down, clutching scrunched-up handkerchiefs and speaking in muffled squeaks to fight back the tears, Dad announced how nice it was to have the old crowd back together. (Dad and his friend had lived in the flat above Mum and her friends in Chelsea.) He added that when Mum was back on her feet again they would all take a trip together, just like old times. I loved my dad's ridiculous optimism and he had no idea just how much his little idiosyncrasies lifted the sombre mood. It was like having a child there who didn't understand what was going on. But really, everyone knew there would never be a 'just like old times' again. It was over.

Later in the afternoon, when all the visitors had gone, I tidied away the last of the cups and glasses and platters of biscuits and shop-bought cake. I was in no mood for baking and G had gone back to the shops for more milk and general supplies. Dad sat napping in the armchair and I looked at him the way I would a puppy, wondering what he dreamed. Did he dream that he was well, that everything was OK? How awful to wake from that and realise it wasn't true. But if he had respite in sleep, then good for him, I would let him sleep some more, so I put a blanket over him and pulled the door tight shut. The nurse team returned to the house as it was getting dark. Mum had not been conscious for hours, and she seemed quite uncomfortable. Her dry mouth was obviously troubling her and she was fidgeting and stirring. She seemed to be dreaming and was reaching out with both hands for something in front of her, as if someone was pulling her up by her arms. The doctor checked her out and then took us downstairs for a chat while the nurses cleaned her up, tidied her hair and changed her nightie.

'OK, this is quite serious, so I understand if you need to stop or talk between yourselves . . .' he began solemnly. 'This is the end. Your mum has only a few days left and we all obviously want to make her as comfortable as possible. She is already on a lot of morphine. The patches are working well, but as she enters the final stages we'll need to help her further. She can't take anything by mouth any more, so the oral morphine can no longer be administered. What I suggest is that we administer a morphine trigger, a kind of continuous injection. If you want us to do this, then we have to move now. It's a complicated process because of the Harold Shipman case. I can prescribe it, but its collection has to be witnessed by someone, so you would both have to pick it up. The night nurse can administer it when she starts later. It will just help her to go peacefully into sleep.'

'So, what are you saying? Are we helping her to die?' Gareth asked slowly, sounding as grave as the doctor. I said nothing, just looked on in concern, my eyes darting between G and the doctor and back again.

'Your mother is already dying. The best thing we can do now is to make her passing as comfortable as possible, but this is completely up to you two.' He paused. 'I also have to ask you both if you want to sign a form on behalf of your mum. It's a form about resuscitation.' We obviously looked scared and rattled. 'Your mum is going to lose consciousness soon. Obviously as doctors we need to try to prolong every patient's life for as long as possible, but in your mum's case it really wouldn't be for very long at all. When she does stop breathing we can resuscitate her and rush her to hospital . . .'

We cut him off almost immediately. 'We don't want that,' we said in unison.

He paused, then continued, 'Or we can let her go here, with you.'

We signed the forms and he signed the prescription for the morphine trigger, hands shaking and signatures barely decipherable. Of all the things you'd never imagine yourself having to do – and there have been a lot of them lately – this was the most surreal. We left Dad still asleep in the armchair and Mum still asleep in her bed. With our aunt making tea and holding the fort, G and I drove to the pharmacy in town. The doctor had called ahead and told them to stay open for us. I am so lucky that my brother and I are such good friends. We feel exactly the same about our parents' care and we have not disagreed about anything really. I cannot imagine going through this with the added agony of arguing with someone over a course of action. We both agreed that Mum should go with some dignity and we didn't want her to have to leave the house again. The last thing we wanted was for her to go through any more upheaval at hospitals, when the chances are the disruption would kill her anyway. We agreed she would have picked this option too. She'd want to be in her own home, lying in her own bed in her own nightie, and with some scented candles and her family nearby. She's going to go out on her own terms.

We went into the pharmacy and produced the prescription slip, which was greeted with solemn faces. The pharmacist and his assistant told the other juniors to go and stand elsewhere while they readied the drugs. Then we all had to sign it: my brother, the two pharmacists and me. I cried and Gareth held me close. I tried to be as quiet as possible, to not draw attention to us. I wanted to be invisible, to stay cocooned in G's safe embrace. I didn't want to look up just in case I saw someone I used to know from school or the pub. I didn't want anyone to see us and feel sorry for us. I just wanted to internalise everything, to just deal with it behind our closed doors. Our family, our issues.

When we got back into the car, G switched the radio on. All I remember of the drive home is being blinded by silent tears while listening to 'Under Pressure' by Queen. My brother remarked on the irony of the song and laughed. It wasn't funny though.

When we got home, both Mum and Dad were awake. My aunt had put Dad to work in the kitchen peeling potatoes for our dinner, he seemed to like being given tasks. Again, he wanted to prove that he was helpful, that he was of use, and he gladly took the instruction and set to work. Mum was lying with her eyes open and she was talking quietly to the nurse, who had stayed on after the other ones had left. She insisted on staying until the night nurse came, saying she would then call her husband to pick her up. It was only later that I realised she had stayed on for about four hours after her shift should have finished. She could have been at home with her own family and she chose to remain with ours, in our hour of need. I know that this is her job, but she went beyond the call of duty and it meant a lot to know that someone else was helping, that someone else cared.

The nurse had already briefed Mum on what was about to happen. Although she was aware of things, she was still very weary and weak. The nurse gave my brother and me a few minutes with her before she began the injection. My brother knelt by her bedside and I lay on top of the bed on her other side, holding her hand.

'Now,' Mum began, 'you kids are to be very good to each other, you hear?'

It was like we were toddlers again, being told off for fighting, which we did, often.

'And you are to look after your father and . . .' She stopped, unable to carry on with her handy parting tips for life. 'I want to thank you so much. I'm so sorry, I don't want to leave you with him, you shouldn't have to do this, to look after and care for . . .'

'We'll be OK,' I cut in. 'You've left us your recipe books!'

It was the only thing I could think of to say that wouldn't make us all cry, but we couldn't ignore the giant deathly elephant in the room. I sat on the bed by her side, chatting softly as her eyes closed and her voice grew distant. I stroked her fingers and thought about how much my hands had started to look like hers. G was on the floor by her other side, kneeling almost in prayer position. I wondered if he was actually praying; it was a bit late for that. She breathed deeper and deeper and looked light, the soft lamp in the corner of the room gently dancing over her cheekbones and eyelashes and I thought she looked beautiful. Despite the awfulness of it, I wanted that moment to last for ever. I knew it would be the last time I would really hear her voice and to really be in her presence. The last time I would have a mummy.

When we got back downstairs, Dad had peeled two whole 2.5kg bags of potatoes. They were immaculate. Fuck knows what we're going to do with them all. We'll be eating mash for months.

## 27th November

The night nurse is here. She's the same lady who has been here all week and she has a kind face and a nice manner. The past few days we've been living in limbo, spending restless nights awaiting the dreaded news, before the dawn comes and brings no respite. I feel like I ought to be accomplishing something during daylight hours but we're all too shattered. If I do sleep then my first thought upon waking is, 'Shit – everyone still alive? We all OK? Right, OK, let's do medicines, feed people, clean people, change people.' If I do venture near slumber my last thought is, 'Shit – everyone still alive?' before the whole process starts again.

When we answered the door to the nurse and welcomed her in, my brother took her coat and she took both our hands in an almost excited way, clamping them together.

'It's going to be tonight, kids, I can feel it in my bones. I've been doing this a very long time and I'm never wrong.'

By this time she was heading for the stairs and up to Mum, while still murmuring, 'Never wrong, never wrong.'

I don't know if that's what they usually do. It's quite weird, but also amusing. I don't know what's wrong with me, because it's actually not funny at all. I feel like I am watching a really obscure comedy and I'm the only person laughing.

I slept in the lounge with my brother again. It was kind of nice in a way, like when you are little and have a sleepover. I remember sometimes on a Friday or Saturday night, Mum would let me sleep in Gareth's room as a treat. I would always feel a little excited about those nights. Sleeping somewhere different to your own bed as a child usually entails fun – it would either mean holidays or being at a friend's house. Obviously, those feelings weren't emulated in the same fashion now. Even though the previous couple of nights had witnessed sleep cruelly dodge me, I fell right into a deep slumber. G had made the bed up for me on the sofa and even put a chocolate on my pillow, just like they do at nice hotels. It was a marshmallow teacake, but the sentiment was there and I enjoyed it immensely, despite eating it merely minutes after having brushed my teeth.

At around 4am, I became aware of someone else in the room. The telly was still on with the sound turned down, and it glowed almost supernaturally in the otherwise pitch-black room. The night nurse was trying to rouse my brother from his peaceful sleep by waggling his big toe. Brave.

'It's happening,' she said in a hushed voice. 'If you want to see her, I'd do it now. I'm sorry.'

My brother turned to me, but he already knew the answer I would give.

'Sorry, bro, no way. I don't want to see her again. I've said everything that I want to say to her. I just can't see her. I just can't.'

I choked and sputtered, the words not feeling like my own.

He kissed my forehead in the same way Mum used to do. 'It's OK, kid, you do whatever feels right. It's your call.'

With that he went upstairs, woke my aunt and they said their goodbyes, muttering private words for her ears only. I sat on the sofa looking up at the ceiling through which I could hear their muffled footsteps where the bed would be. When they eventually came back down, tear-stained and shaky, I felt like a childish drop-out for not going the last leg with them.

Gareth said Mum was making funny noises, like her breathing was stopping. The so-called death rattle. We let Dad sleep, as we didn't want to confuse him further, not yet. Then the three of us made tea and sat in the front room watching telly, well not really watching, more staring blankly at *Takeshi's Castle* with the sound turned down. Just as we were silently watching crazy Japanese folk falling into a dirty castle moat, the nurse reappeared.

She came bearing the inevitable news that I had dreaded hearing for days.

'I'm so sorry . . . your mother has passed.'

Only when she delivered those fateful words, words that would change my life for ever, I didn't feel as bad as I thought I would. For weeks I had cried at the thought of being told of Mum's death, but honestly, at that moment, it just felt like cold fact.

The nurse held my hand. 'You leave everything to me. I will look after her now. Do you want to come up and see her?'

'Uh, no, not really,' I said, almost laughing.

'She is very peaceful,' she added, as if that might convince me to see someone who was no longer alive. I could tell I was pulling that weird face that makes people uncomfortable.

My brother kindly intervened. 'I would like to see her and I'll wake Dad,' he said.

We all knew that this needed to be done, but as usual it was my brave brother who made the move. My aunt seconded the motion and went upstairs to fetch him. Dad padded into the living room with fuzzy hair and crumpled pyjamas. He was still dazed by sleep and rubbing his eyes like a toddler.

'Sit down, Dad,' I said gently. I took his hand and knelt in front of him. 'Dad, you know how Mum has been very ill, yes?'

Dad nodded and I could tell that he already knew what was coming. I took a deep breath. 'Mum passed away just a little while ago.'

He looked sad, but there was no shock or an immediate reaction.

'OK, oh, that's very bad news,' he said, starting to weep softly.

'Would you like to see her, Dad?' I asked, giving his hands what I hoped was a reassuring squeeze.

'Um, yes, I want to see my wife. I'll have to get dressed then, which hospital is she at?'

'No, Dad, she's here, she's in bed. Do you remember? That's why you have been sleeping in the spare room. We'll take you upstairs if you really want to see her.'

As I spoke, I passed his hand into my brother's.

He led him upstairs, my aunt in tow. I sat downstairs on my own and wondered what it was like up there. I know she didn't look any different. She couldn't, could she? But I stand by my decision not to see her, as I truly think that it would have haunted me. I prefer to always think of my mum as I saw her last, sleeping peacefully and gently squeezing my hand as I told her that I loved her for the last time.

As I got upset, she had whispered, 'I'm just your daft old mum.'

I hope she knows that I still love her and always will. Just because I can't say it to her doesn't mean I don't think it. I believe that I love her more with every passing minute. Right then, as I stood in the kitchen clutching my cold cup of tea, I felt that she was there. I could almost see her, too. She was in her pink cotton nightdress and I could smell her face cream, feel her hands on my shoulders and hear her whisper. I can't really explain it, but it felt like she was walking around the house. I didn't feel spooked out or scared, but I truly felt she was there. My aunt came back into the kitchen and held me.

'I don't want her to go,' I sobbed, and my tears dampened the collar of her dressing gown.

After some discussion, we decided to send Dad back to bed. We took the line that we were all going to get some more sleep. He duly obliged and trod back up the stairs alone. He was now a single man, a widower.

The nurse had called the funeral directors for us and she tidied up Mum's things, straightened her nightdress, brushed her hair while we waited for them to come for her.

Now, when I said that I could feel Mum's presence in the kitchen, I do largely understand that this often happens to people when they lose someone – it doesn't mean that it's true.

I realise that I may have concocted this ridiculous notion to comfort myself and that there was nothing tangible to suggest that my mum's spirit had manifested to do a tour of the house. However, what happened next was so clear that I will never ever forget it. Not till the day I die. My brother, my aunt and I sat silently in the lounge, drinking more tea, red-eyed and fragile; it was just about an hour after Mum had passed. I honestly can find no explanation for what followed. Suddenly, all the lights went off, like we were at a theatre and a play was about to start. They kind of dimmed, for a few seconds at least, then came back up again. I looked towards my aunt, then Gareth, but before I had the chance to question it, it happened again, and it wasn't just the lights, it was the TV, too, and the lights out in the kitchen. They came back on again to full strength and stayed on. We looked at each other in disbelief, speechless and confused.

'Am I on drugs, or did that just happen?'

My aunt concurred that no, I was not hallucinating.

My brother had lost the power of speech but did make some gurgling noises.

'How strange,' my aunt said, clearly shaken. 'I don't . . . I don't understand, perhaps it was a power cut.'

Just then the nurse came back into the room. 'Right, I tidied up all your mum's stuff and have bagged up all the medicine, but I'll take you through what to do with that later because I will come back to talk to you all. You all look very shocked – I think you need to try and get some rest, easier said than done, I know . . .' She trailed off and looked down to her feet.

'Did the lights just go out upstairs?' my brother asked. 'We think we may have had a power cut.'

'Ooh no, love, I don't think so. I had them switched on in Mum's room so I could see what I was doing – they're still on. Is everything OK?'

Now, I don't know what happened with the lights in the house, perhaps it was Mum saying goodbye, though I don't feel that it's really her style, she knows how easily I scare. I don't know whether it was death, or an energy, or what, but something happened in this house, it was so clear and the three of us know that we will never, ever forget it.

More time passed. I don't really recall exact events but I do remember the funeral directors coming and saying that they would take Mum, that they would look after her, and that they would put her in the chapel and that she would be OK with them. I believe them. They seem nice. I went outside for a cigarette then, as I didn't want to see them take her from her home; the sad inelegance of a proud woman exiting the nest she feathered in a wooden box.

After I came back from my cigarette, one of the funeral directors was saying goodbye to my brother and aunt at the door. Then the three of us stood in the living room watching his dark shadow floating down the pathway and out into the eerie early dawn. We heard the van start up and pull away from the house. Then all the lights went out again, for about ten seconds this time. None of us said a word. Mum was gone.

### 28th November

Mum died yesterday.

### 29th November

Mum died the day before yesterday.

### 30th November

Mum died two days ago.

### 1st December

Today people start opening their advent calendars. Not me; today just marks another day I have to tell my dad that he is now a widower. Or not. I can't bear doing it any more. The past couple of days have been a blur of tears, cooking food then throwing the food in the bin, then turning the telly on and off again. Of avoiding people and sitting outside in the cold smoking fags, before Dad comes out with ridiculous shit about being the man of the house and how he needs to get all our affairs in order. Within the hour he asks for Mum again and we go through the disbelief, the tears, the anger or the sheer indifference.

I'm fucking sick of it, so today I went for Christmas lunch at a hotel with Mum's friends. It had been arranged for a long time and was one of their regular girls' get-togethers. They were going to cancel it, but I asked them if they could go ahead and whether I could join in Mum's place. I know she wouldn't have wanted to waste the money and they may have had to pay a fee, as it was so close to Christmas. It was a stupid thing to concern myself with, but that was my mum talking – the frugal Scot through and through. I thought it seemed like a nice thing to do, so we all went together. I haven't really cried yet. I haven't felt like it – everyone's been really nice and it's been kind of overwhelming. A friend of mine who lost her father a year ago has been really good with me, as well as honest. She took me to the supermarket the other day in an attempt to cheer me up. (The supermarket is an odd choice, I know, but nothing seems to make sense right now. Plus, she is kind of mental herself, and I mean mental in the most amazing way.) She told me that when her dad died she didn't feel sad at first. In fact, in the first few weeks she actually felt rather elated. There was such an outpouring of support and love in the form of cards and well-wishes that it was difficult to feel down. She warned me that her darkest period came after all this ended.

'Great, I'll look forward to that then,' I said grimly.

So anyway, I went to the lunch with Mum's friends. It was a nice enough hotel, about five miles from the house, and I had actually showered and blow-dried my hair properly, I put on make-up, a process I rather enjoyed, and looking and feeling presentable almost boosted my spirits. I wore a floral tea dress and one of Mum's cashmere shawls with a brooch on the shoulder. They had all waited for me in the lobby area and while G couldn't face them (understandable, he was leaving that duty to me), they surrounded me like a warm swarm, hugging and loving. Like when you see penguins huddle together on wildlife documentaries, the youngest and weakest hidden in the middle, protected. Most of them sobbed through the meal, which I found quite distracting. I also worried about what people on neighbouring tables must have thought, a group of women weeping under elaborate tinsel and wreaths of fake mistletoe. At one point one of them scrunched up yet another tear-soaked tissue and placed it behind her atop the nativity display. I'm sure my mum wouldn't have cried, she would have told people to pull themselves together. It was rather nice, though, being with them all. I found it comforting. I'm not sure what they all thought of me, do I look like I am coping? Do I look like I am grieving? I think they pity me, and I don't really like that. I know it comes from a loving and motherly place, but sympathy is really not what I want. I'm not that good at reading the thoughts of others at the moment. I'm confused by my own.

I explained to Mum's friends about the funeral plans. The local church first, then the crematorium, then the wake at a country hotel. I told them how at some point I wanted them to come round to the house and choose something of Mum's to keep; a scarf, a piece of jewellery, or something from her vast collection of ornamental elephants – her favourite animal. She had amassed her collection from far and wide. There were pieces sourced in Africa and those that friends and family had bought for her over the years. I really don't know what I'm going to do with all her stuff. Mum's friends seemed to like the idea of picking something that belonged to her. I would rather her belongings were somewhere they might be cherished and loved rather than just being thrown away or gathering dust in a charity shop. Alone.

Gareth picked me up from the lunch and we went to the funeral directors' on the way home. Such a fun-packed day. It's kind of like planning a wedding, but really shit.

They ask you all sorts of things you never really want to think about, such as what music you would want to play at the funeral of your loved one so that each time you hear it, for the rest of your life, you'll be reduced to a horrid weepy mess and will never be able to listen to that song/artist/genre ever again. As Mum had been aware that the end was nigh for her, she had made a few suggestions. We went with a piece of music by the composer John Barry from the film *Out of Africa*. They had spent so much of their life in Kenya, especially Dad – through his work. Gareth had been born in Nairobi, and they had loved it there, a raw and real landscape with few of the complications of western civilisations. They also asked us about readings, etc., but the vicar had said she would come to see us this evening and we would decide all that then. I didn't really want to see the sodding vicar, I just wanted to eat fish and chips on my own. Mind you, the vicar is really nice, a female vicar – how modern! – and we have known her a long time. She used to be the local hairdresser, she gave me my first perm that made me look like Kevin Keegan, not intentional, but it went with the times. I don't think she does hair any more, just church stuff. Anyway, I do like that she will be looking after Mum's day as she knows Mum and Dad (knew Mum, do I say that yet?).

The funeral directors' place was right by my old school and we always used to joke when we walked past it about how many dead people were in there. Our mum was now one of them. Which is really weird. Nice guys, though, the funeral directors.

Such a macabre career. In between selecting flowers, coffins, cars, we couldn't help but ask childish, ghoulish questions.

My brother went first. 'So, uh, like, how many people do you have here?'

In his baritone Welsh lilt, one of the directors said, 'Well, myself, my brother, my two sons and another full-time member of staff and . . .'

'No, dead ones,' Gareth corrected, trying not to giggle.

The funeral director looked shocked. 'Oh, well, it obviously varies . . .' He tailed off and looked to his desk.

'You must see some really weird stuff, though, right?' I said.

The funeral director leant over his desk and lowered his voice. He was almost smiling now. 'Ooooh yes, my dear, I couldn't even begin to tell you . . .'

Before I could ask him to elaborate he snapped his folder shut, making us jump and signalling the end of that line of questioning. 'Well, then, you two, I shall come round again in the next two days with the final draft for the Order of Service and we can run through the whole process. Please don't worry about a thing, we'll help you through.'

On our way out he smiled at us and shook our hands tenderly. I thought he was a nice man.

Back in the car, my brother and I continued our creepy conversation.

'I reckon they must see all sorts of mental shit,' I said. 'Do you think they ever get scared?'

'Yeah, but I bet the money helps. Fuck me, funerals aren't cheap.'

'To be honest, if I had to deal with dead people all day I would want a lot of money, too. You know we have to pick out an outfit for Mum, to give to them? Isn't that just fucking creepy? Someone dressing your dead mother.'

'Stop it. I think I'm going to puke. That's really rank.'

'Yeah, weird.'

'Really fucking weird.'

We drove home listening to Radiohead's 'Everything In Its Right Place'. Except it wasn't.

## 3rd December

A little lesson in what not to say to children in moments of grief. Our wonderful neighbour came round to offer her condolences. She was very tearful and so sincere; it's weird to see other people cry about your family, especially when your own tears won't come. But she did make us smile. In an attempt to explain to her five-year-old son what had happened to Aunty Marge next door, she'd sat him down the previous evening and explained that Aunty Marge had been ill and she had gone up into the sky to live. She pointed up at the twinkling stars and said that she was up there smiling down on us.

The boy's wide-eyed retort?
'How'd she get up there then? Rocket?'
Priceless!

## 6th December

Funeral day. Why are they so close to the person's
death? It's cruel, isn't it? You haven't even got used
to the idea of them not being there any more, and
then you have to stick them in the ground or in a fire.
There's not even time to think, or hurt, or breathe,
and it's just so cruel. I thought I was OK. I didn't
feel bad when I woke up this morning, but then all
the family were around and I felt like the baby again.
I probably acted like a bit of a brat, too. I couldn't
find anything to wear, which seems like such a stupid
and inconsequential thing to get het up about, but I
didn't want people to think I looked a mess. I wanted
them to think I'm OK, because I am OK. I think.

I woke Dad and reminded him what today was. I
don't think he gets it 100 per cent, which is a bit of
a blessing, really. He was quiet and compliant, not
trying to take over or anything, just sitting where we
showed him to and keeping his shit together. I was
dreading other people's reactions to him; again, I
don't want pity – not for me or him. He is proud.

I felt sick when the car arrived, but then it was
all right. We all got into it and got to the church.
Well, only just. The whole road was taken up with

cars. The church is at the end of a narrow little lane, which means you're in trouble if you meet another car coming the other way. When we rounded the corner at the top of the lane, I choked up. One of the farmers had very kindly opened his field for parking and it was full.

The cavalcade proceeded slowly down the lane for nearly a quarter of a mile. People were walking towards the church and they stopped, turned and bowed their heads as we passed. The church car park was full and there were people outside the church who couldn't fit inside. It was full to the brim. All here for my mum.

We had arranged for a bagpiper to play Mum into the church. She always liked the bagpipes, they reminded her of bonny Scotland. I don't know anyone else who actually likes the sound, other than the Scottish. As the directors were getting Mum's coffin ready to come out of the car, we had a quick chat with the bagpiper.

'Don't worry about the weather,' he said to us. 'It'll brighten up now. The sun will shine for her, trust me.'

He gave a smile and a little wink and, as we turned to the church, there was the slightest glint of blue sky. The day was blustery and cool, the weather seemed like it didn't know what to do, whether to be stormy and petulant, or brooding and sulking. Dad didn't ask about carrying the coffin and I'm glad; Gareth did it along with Uncle Eddie, Mum's younger brother, Uncle Jim, Aunty Judith's husband, and my cousin Paul. What an awful thing to do, to carry a coffin containing someone you love. I got the easy job of walking in with Dad. Just before we went into the church he took my hand in his and then linked it through the crook of his arm and told me that everything was going to be OK. He knew what was going on, right then, and I wanted to believe him with all my heart.

As we went into the church I felt a lurch of sadness that this could have been a much happier occasion; Dad could have been walking me down the aisle on my wedding day, all happiness and smiles with Mum waiting in a fancy hat. She would never see me get married, she would never meet her grandchildren, she would never get to know what happens next. I threw up a little in my mouth and swallowed it as everyone in the congregation turned to look at us. I just stared at my feet and made sure that they kept moving, one in front of the other, in front of the other.

I'd decided to speak at the church. I used a book I'd had made for Mum's 60th birthday. It was like a *This is Your Life* book – a big red album full of pictures from her childhood, her friends and family, important milestones and things she loved. I can't even really recall what I said, but I guess it was OK. People smiled, some even laughed. I didn't feel that bad when I had to stand up. I have never had a fear of public speaking, talking is one of the things I can do and I felt better once I was sort of in charge of the situation. The *Out of Africa* song was so fitting in the end. This was a place where Mum and Dad had felt happy, young and free.

We then went on to the crematorium, where my brother read a poem. It seemed as if there were even more people there than in the church. Do funeral processions pick up more people as they trundle along their merry way – like some sort of macabre Pied Piper? I tried not to think about it. When they played the final bit of music and Mum's coffin rattled off behind the curtains, I could hear people sobbing. But oddly enough, I didn't cry.

By the time we got to the hotel, I was exhausted. I was tired of keeping an eye on Dad, like a nervous mother watchful of her naughty toddler, but he was good (well, he was mental in parts) and mostly just stuck by our side. We had nice food, some cake and a little booze. All in all, it wasn't the awful day I had expected. Is it bad to think that?

I'd worried Dad might want to do a speech and then not be able to, but fortunately he didn't mention it. At the wake, though, he did seem to lose the meaning of what the day was for. He seemed to really perk up; maybe it was the energy of having so many people about, I guess he hadn't been around that many people (especially those he knew) for a long time, so it must have been really disorientating. He said to a group of Mum's friends how lucky he felt that so many people had come out to help him celebrate his retirement. They made a hasty retreat, obviously feeling uncomfortable, which made me a little angry. After that, while I was having a cigarette outside, he apparently did a little solo waltz across the middle of the hall floor, as people stood solemnly drinking cups of tea. He tried to grab the hand of an old neighbour and loudly asked the congregation, 'Why aren't you dancing? Come on – everybody should be dancing!'

When my brother told me this I laughed, cried and then laughed again. Apparently people were aghast. Fuck them! I would have danced with him.

At one point, I found Dad sitting in a corner with one of my friend's little daughters on his lap. She is only four and they were both holding one of her dolls. I slid silently up to stand just behind them, unnoticed. The little girl asked Dad how he was doing.

'Well, I'm fine,' he said. 'I do love a party!'

'Is this a party for you, then?' she asked.

'Yes, love, I think so, it must be.'

'Don't you know?' the little girl giggled.

Dad giggled too. 'Oh, my dear. I don't know much of anything these days.'

'Is there cake?'

'Well, I hope so. I like cake. Do you like cake?'

'Yes. And pop.'

'Well, shall we go and see if we can find my birthday cake then?'

'Is it your birthday?' the girl asked, wide-eyed.

'Yes, love, I think so, it must be.'

They stood up, he took her little hand in his and they walked together to the buffet table. I was happy that my friend saw absolutely no risk in leaving her daughter with the man who had looked after her when she was that age. I was also happy that my dad had found company with the one person in that whole hotel who didn't judge him or pity him or patronise him.

Apart from his Fred Astaire moment, everyone said Dad seemed and looked really well. I suppose he did, if you weren't looking too closely. They also asked us all how we were coping. What are you meant to say to that? Especially to people you don't know that well? You could opt for, 'I feel like my heart has actually left my body and there is a gaping, great big black hole where once there was love. I can't sleep or eat or think. In fact, right now I am wondering how I'm managing to stand up straight. I am unsure if I can hold a rational conversation and nothing, nothing, is certain. I think I might die, just stop living. You don't matter to me and I don't matter to me. What has happened is so absolutely insurmountable that the only person who could make it right is in a wooden box in a church.'

Or. . .

'Yeah, I'm fine. I'll be fine.'

I went with the second option. Obviously.

Then you get The Arm Rub from people and The Sad-Eyed Smile, where they don't actually open their mouths.

After the people had all queued up to touch our arms again and give us The Sad-Eyed Smile, we all went home, to a home that Mum no longer shared. There was plenty of food left over and I decided to take it with us. Dad wanted his 'birthday cake' and we got some board games out. Even Dad wanted to join in, and we played Scrabble. It was a really old set, maybe 30 years old. The board was tattered and torn, the letters faded and the box ragged and worn. It smelled of family history, of good times and joy. Opening the box let out almost three decades of memories.

Every time Dad picked out a letter, he said, 'Ha ha, look at this now, kids, eh? You see how faded the letters are? That's how often we played this! All the flipping time! Ah, this is good, a nice family game of Scrabble.'

He proceeded to show us all of his letters to prove his point. We would take our turns then prompt Dad to pick more letters. This was his cue to repeat his mini monologue.

We laughed along with him. It was very sweet and endearing. Dad made us endless cups of tea. Gareth, who doesn't do hot drinks, accepted them anyway, letting them get cold before chucking them in the plant behind the table. I swear to God that plant will die this week, too. And then we took our own Scrabble turns. By the time we reached the end of the game, Dad's interest had waned and he left the table to use the bathroom before bed. He kissed us on the head, told us he loved us very much and thanked us for a lovely day.

We looked at each other, bemused, but only a little. As Dad plodded up the stairs and we cleared the table, I looked down at the pad and paper where we'd been keeping the score. Dad had won by 58 points.

## 7th December

The lessons you learn in life: an urn full of ashes is a very heavy thing. We had to go back to the funeral directors' to pick it up. It's quite big, like a vase, and it really weighs a ton, far more than I had expected. But then I don't really know what I had expected. Carrying my mother's remains in a pot isn't something I tended to spend much time pondering.

We left Dad in the car when we went into the funeral parlour. I didn't want to freak him out . . . whether he would have understood where he was or not was another matter. I kept looking out of the window to check he was OK. He was making silly faces and actions, as if he was playing a one-man game of charades. The funeral director asked how he was. He was fully aware of the situation and, as I watched my dad attempt to disco-dance in the front seat with his seatbelt still on, I smiled and said he was fine. They handed Mum over, together with a small brown envelope, which had her wedding ring in it. I held that, too. Gareth drove us home with Dad next to him in the front and me and Mum, in her urn, in the back.

'What you got there then, love?' Dad asked. We had agreed it was best not to tell him and to keep the urn in its box, out of sight.

'It's, uh, just . . . uh, um, shall we go home via the lakes on top of the mountain?'

Distraction tactics – it's not really lying, right? So we drove home the long way, with Mum resting heavy on my knees. At the top of the mountain we got out and walked slowly around the lido. Dad had his hands clasped behind his back, in the way old men do. His tweed flat cap was perched regally on his head as he took deep, loud inhalations of fresh, Welsh mountain air. The view up there is exactly what you picture when people talk of the Welsh valleys: miles and miles of rough grassy undulations speckled with little rows of terraced miners' houses, rocky outcrops and bare patches indicating locations of now-barren mines, Cordell's *Rape of the Fair Country* clear for all to see. There's a stillness up here, far above the towns in the valleys below; a working man's majesty set to the soundtrack of the melodic murmur of bleating sheep. If you closed your eyes and surrendered yourself to their lowing you could almost hear them humming 'Calon Lân'. Meanwhile, I fretted about the car being broken into and someone stealing my dead mother's ashes.

When we got home, we decided to put Mum on her bookcase in the bedroom. We left the urn in its box, so it wouldn't attract any attention. After that, we discussed sleeping arrangements. I knew I didn't want to sleep in a bed that someone had died in, and I couldn't imagine Dad would either, especially as this was his wife. We asked him, delicately of course, if he would prefer to sleep in the second bedroom from now on, and he agreed. It was a solemn moment but one in which I think he had complete lucidity.

And so it was that Mum and Dad's bedroom sat empty at night. Dad slept in my brother's room, my brother slept in my room and I slept in the lounge. Except I didn't really sleep. None of us did.

### 8th December

The house is lonely and the house is cold. The house is full of her things, her smell . . . her. And him. He asked me again this morning where she was. I'm tired of telling the truth and I am tired of breaking his heart, so I lie to him, and I don't care what anyone thinks about that. The morning after the funeral he knew; he was inconsolable, heavy sobs emanating from his bed, cries so deep and tortured I thought he might throw up. He didn't want company or consolation, he wanted solitude. But by lunchtime he thought she was at work and asked me if I would be staying for tea before heading back to university.

When I woke this morning, I noticed his bedroom door was open and his bedclothes had been thrown aside, as if he'd risen in a hurry. He wasn't in the bathroom or the kitchen or the lounge, and the back door was open. I looked further down the garden and saw the shed was unlocked, its door ajar. Hurriedly wrapping my dressing gown fiercely around me against the bracing chill, I tiptoed down the path, fearing the worst and calling out for Dad, softly but urgently. As I neared the shed, I heard rustling.

'Hello?' Dad said.

He was crouched beneath his long-abandoned tool bench, riffling through old crates.

My heart fluttered with relief, thank fuck for that!

'Morning, Dad. What you up to?'

'Oh, God, love, thank God you've arrived. I'm really starting to panic.'

Dad stood up and raised a dirty, sweaty hand to his fuzzy bed-head. His tired, old, pale, striped pyjamas were ruffled and creased and his look was one of sheer confusion.

'It's your mum, she's been missing for weeks now. I can't find her anywhere. I've called the police and everything. I think they've taken her!'

Dad was trembling, his voice breaking.

Before I even got to who would have taken her, whether he had actually called the police and why he thought the tool shed would hold the key to her disappearance, I took his hand.

'Why don't we just go back up to the house and have a cup of tea and then we can sort this all out, eh?'

In that moment there was nothing else I could do, I would not break his heart again and I would not break mine further, the little shattered pieces I had left only just holding out. All I could hope for was that this momentary sadness would not last, that his brain would zone out again to some fake happiness, some invented normality – it was easier for him and thus for me.

I let him put his arm around me and we walked over the crisp, frozen lawn and up the cold, concrete steps. By the time the kettle was on and the hot steam was clouding up the chilled kitchen windows, the whole scenario was a distant memory . . . at least for Dad.

## 9th December

Dad went out with his carer today and my brother and I went through some of Mum's things. We didn't really want to, but we felt we ought to at least do something, otherwise it was as if we were avoiding the whole situation. We held the box with her urn in it and spoke to her, more in a jokey way, although I can understand how it may sound a bit sinister. To be fair, this whole carry-on is a bit sinister, but I'm so far removed from real life right now that I couldn't give a fuck.

I picked up Mum's jewellery box, and I could smell her when I opened it. I felt like a little girl again and remembered when I would sneak into my parents' room and try on Mum's necklaces, as if I was a grown-up. I knew exactly the necklace I was looking for on this trip down memory lane – a double-layer crystal droplet with a huge clasp that did up at the nape of the neck. I put it on. It looked great with sweatpants and my old Aerosmith T-shirt. I touched it to my skin and I felt like her, which made me smile.

'See, that's the shit thing right there,' my brother said, from his seated position on the windowsill. 'You get good stuff like that . . . stuff you can wear every day and be closer to her. What do I get?'

'Well, you can have a necklace, too, if you want,' I giggled.

We spent ages at the bottom of Mum and Dad's bed finding memories . . . not just her trinkets, but what she'd kept of us: first teeth, Mother's Day cards, school reports (Gareth's were better than mine). It wasn't just memories of our mother we uncovered, but her memories of us, and the things she cherished. These, in turn, became our memories again.

## 10th December

Woke up this morning and panicked about Dad; he is always my first thought and always my last. Will he ask about Mum today? Will he be aware? Will he be angry? Will he be violent? What can I cook him? Turns out I didn't need to think about that last question. I stuck my head into his bedroom and he wasn't there (more panic sets in) but his bed was made (some days he remembers, some days he doesn't) so I hurried down the stairs to find him sitting at the dining table staring at some brochures, fully dressed in trousers, shirt, tie and pullover, ready for action.

'All right, Da?'

'Hello, love, didn't know you were staying over!'

He had the phone in hand and was looking carefully through what I could now see were Chinese take-away menus.

'I thought I would get some dinner in, look here . . .' He waved the garish card menus. 'These folk say they deliver, not all the way from China obviously!' He laughed, slapping his thigh. 'But just from town, that's good of them, isn't it? Anyway, I think I've got this number in all wrong as I can't get through.'

I haven't been aware of Dad eating Chinese food since we were actually in China for his work, many many years ago. He has never expressed any interest in the cuisine, and especially not in having it delivered! I don't know why that was my focus, and not the fact that he was attempting to order sweet and sour pork balls at eight in the morning.

## 16th December

This morning began as it usually did. I woke up, checked on Dad, found his arse sticking out of the bottom of the wardrobe, had the usual conversation with him about looking for Mum and only momentarily pondered why he would look for her in the wardrobe. To be honest, I don't know how it started or why. I lost my temper . . . I know I shouldn't have. I snapped at him about something trivial and he snapped right back.

'I will fucking end you, do you hear me?' he snarled, with his face right up to mine. 'I don't know who you are, or why you're here, but I want you out of this house. THIS IS MY HOUSE! Do you hear me, you little fucking piece of shit?'

When he reached for my throat, I ducked and scarpered, darting down the corridor and leaping down the stairs. I slipped on the bottom few and twisted my ankle. Panicking and sweating, I hurriedly limped through to the living room to pick up the phone to try to reach my brother, who had gone into town for some shopping. I wasn't going back upstairs. You know when you see people in films who can think really quickly and plan an escape route? Well, that must be 100 per cent poetic licence because I ummed and ahhed for ages and fumbled with the phone. I could hear Dad coming down the stairs, getting closer.

'Where are you, you fucking little thief?' he yelled. 'You think you can come into my house and rob my things? I'm going to kill you, you hear me?'

I ducked behind the sofa and dropped the phone as he came into the room. I could see that he was holding a carving knife. He looked towards the window and then backed away, walking through the dining room and into the kitchen. I could see his feet from under the sofa. He had his slippers on the wrong way round. I couldn't make it to the front door, as he would see me and block my route, and I couldn't get out of the back door, as I would have to pass him. I was trapped.

Then I heard him put the kettle on and mutter to himself. I prayed for this to be a moment where he would forget. I could hear him rummaging around in the kitchen drawers. Someone knocked on the door. He didn't move. The person knocked again. He walked to the front of the house and opened the heavy old door, which creaked.

'Hi there! You all right?'

It was the next-door neighbour.

'Hello there, love!' My dad's voice was all soft and fatherly, not mad and murderous. 'How can I help you today?'

'We, uh, we just heard some noise next door and wondered if you were OK . . . Why, why do you have a carving knife in your hand?'

'Well, funnily enough, I've just found a burglar in my house, so right now I'm trying to smoke the little fucker out,' Dad declared, rather proudly.

The neighbour had seen me in the garden just half an hour earlier. I prayed she would know it was me, and that I needed help.

'OK . . . can I help you?'

She knew, but she was also scared. I could hear it in her voice. 'Why don't I come inside?'

'No, it's OK,' Dad said. 'I'm just going to execute her. That's what you have to do these days, isn't it? Protect yourself, protect your family. My wife is ill upstairs in our bed and I'll be damned if someone's going to come in here . . .'

He went on. I could tell the neighbour was trying to stall him. I had to make a break for it. While he was facing the street I could dart to the other side of the dining table and out into the garden. Once there I could run over the lawn and climb the wall into next-door's garden. I went for it, snaking across the floor while hoping that the neighbour would keep Dad talking. If he came for me with that knife, I knew I wouldn't escape. I crawled to the back door. Shit, it was locked! I reached up to the corner of the table, hands shaking as I scrabbled and searched for the key. I fumbled with the lock then slid the door open and rolled out onto the patio, getting to my feet and sprinting down the garden before hurling myself up over the wall and cutting my face on the brickwork. There was no sign of Dad. I lay on the lawn in next-door's garden, panting for breath in the cold, damp grass. I rolled over again and climbed their wall into the next garden. Then I climbed another wall into a side street. I couldn't go back. I had no phone, no wallet, no money and, looking down, no shoes.

I hid by the side of the house. The front of our door was just visible and I could see that Dad had gone back inside. There was every chance I could just waltz back in as if nothing had happened . . . every chance he wouldn't notice or remember. But there was also every chance he was still brandishing the carving knife and baying for the blood of the burglar.

I didn't want to risk it. But then what if he was about to harm himself? I couldn't go next door, as he would see me.

Despondent, I walked the long way away from the house, trudging up the hill and round the block, down the hill and across town, up the other side of the valley to my friend Kate's house, slopping through the damp streets with no shoes on. She had a young baby and I knew she would be at home. Plus, she'd been such a good support throughout this whole ordeal so far. She opened the door to my tear-stained, bloodied face and my frozen, sodden feet.

Together, we called the local authorities and the Alzheimer's Support care staff. I was advised not to return to the house. They told me that I was not to put myself in a position of danger, as I could easily be harmed. If that happened the police would have to be involved and Dad might be arrested. We called my brother who laughed before crying. It reminded me of the time he crashed his car, back when we were teenagers. He had just passed his test and we'd been out for a spin. He was coming down the driveway towards the house, a little fast, I thought, but I didn't say. Then I suddenly realised he wasn't stopping. The car buckled into the side of the house and the bonnet scrunched up like paper. Though both unharmed, we were totally shocked. We got out of the car and looked at the mess we'd made. Then we looked at each other and cracked up, bending over double and hooting with laughter. Dad had heard the commotion and felt the impact of the car hitting the house. He opened the front door to see his selfish, stupid little children in hysterics. After he'd taken a long look at us, he walked out the back of the house and disappeared. It was then we began to cry.

And so I stayed here, at my friend's house. By the time my brother got back to the house, Dad had apparently made himself cheese on toast and two cups of tea. Gareth picked up the carving knife from the side table by the sofa and then collected all the sharp knives and put them in the boot of his car. Dad didn't mention Mum, but he did say that I wouldn't be bothering them any more, that he had seen to it that I would leave them alone. I had been 'dealt with'.

### 17th December

We stuck by our plan that it was best for me to stay away, at least for a while. G brought me a few things; jumpers, shampoo, make-up, a phone charger, cigarettes, my diary.

Meanwhile, I watched my friend Kate's new baby writhe around the living-room floor, I played with her dog, read books by the fireplace, ate her lovely, home-cooked vegetarian food and marvelled at this normal and blissful domestic existence. It felt nice and I wondered whether I might find such peace one day. But when I went to bed I cried and experienced only guilt and horror.

## 19th December

Dad went out with his carer again today, so I took the opportunity to go back to the house and collect some more stuff. Now that the house is solely occupied by men, it feels different, even though nothing has changed. I collected a change of clothes, underwear, shampoo and some money. I also had time for a cup of tea and a chat with Mum's ashes. I sat in the old captain's chair by the bookcase in their room and rested the urn in my lap as I looked out of the window and over the town.

I remembered the night she died. I remembered my brother standing in the bay window downstairs, tutting as he watched two lovers stumble past, drunken hand in drunken hand, giggling and chatting, kissing and laughing.

'How can they carry on like that? It's nearly four in the morning and there's someone DYING in here,' he exclaimed.

'They're not to know, are they?' I whispered, as he walked off to the back of the house. And it made me think. They probably went home and had sex that night. Maybe they even made a baby. And somewhere close by a baby may have been born. People were sleeping, watching telly, kissing, crying, rowing, working, making up, breaking up, having a good time, having a bad time. Life was going on around us as Mum's ended. And that didn't make me mad, it comforted me.

My tea had gone cold and my time was running out. I kissed Mum, put her back on the shelf and made a hasty departure before Dad got home.

## 20th December

I met my brother in town. He's a mess. He can't cope. Dad is driving him mad. He won't sleep or eat. He keeps asking where Mum and me are. Having witnessed our struggle, and in light of Dad's violent outbursts, the local authority has offered to arrange a temporary respite care stay at a home in a nearby town. It's a rational, if heart-breaking, option, and it's one that neither of us really want to take. We sat together in Wetherspoons, drinking soda water and hating ourselves.

'How bad has he been really?' I asked.

'I always reckoned I could care for him up until the point he couldn't go to the toilet without assist-ance,' he replied.

'And has he reached that point?'

'No, which is why I feel like such a failure. I can't even look after my own fucking father,' he said, his voice wavering with self-hatred.

'You aren't a failure and you know that. For fuck's sake, I couldn't look after him.'

'Yeah, but he did try to kill you. And that's kind of bad, isn't it?'

'Guess so,' I replied. We almost laughed.

Since Mum died, Dad has gone downhill rapidly. I understand that for Alzheimer's sufferers, changes in routine and security can hugely affect their decline, and this has most certainly happened in Dad's case. He is constantly disorientated, has very little appetite and barely speaks. We have been prescribed more medication for him, especially antidepressants, which are obviously just numbing his senses and putting him in some sort of damp bubble of solitude.

We've agreed to a temporary 10-day stay in a respite home after Christmas, just so that we can get some rest. We've both been intent on internalising our family 'issue'. We thought we could cope, we would cope . . . we would handle this ourselves. But, of course, we can't. We are failing our father, failing each other, and we are also failing ourselves.

Since I became a refugee I've roamed from friend's house to friend's house. Their generosity is wavering now, though, in favour of their close families. It's Christmas after all, and this is totally understandable. But I know where I can go.

## 24th December

Yesterday I took a taxi all the way to the station and boarded the big train to Paddington. I had a bottle of vodka with me, which I drank neat. I didn't even care enough to disguise it. A mother moved her two young children away from me on the train, as I slurringly showed my ticket to the inspector. From Paddington, I took the bus to Camden and went straight to the pub. My friends greeted me, by which time I was already very pissed. I propped up the railing outside the pub, chain-smoking in the cold night with my coat and scarf wrapped tight around me. People worried, I know they did, but I was too far gone to even lie to them and pretend I was fine. They knew better than to ask or try to intervene. I vaguely remember getting bundled into a taxi and taken back to Candy and Emma's house, where the party went on around me as I drifted in and out of consciousness.

This morning, they packed for home, to spend Christmas with their families. I had many invitations for the festive period, but all I wanted was to be alone. My brother was still with Dad, so I sat and got high on my own, in the cold and empty house. I consumed paltry party food for one purchased from the cheapest supermarket. I drank, I smoked, I mourned, I wallowed and I loathed.

## *25th December*

My brother called. Apparently, Dad has a hernia the size of Guernsey. He thought it would be a nice Christmas present to show him over breakfast. It's so bad they have spent most of Christmas Day at the hospital, with pissed-off staff who would rather be at home with their loved ones than prodding and poking my bulging old man. My brother told the doctors about Dad's situation and the fact he was about to go into respite care. They now don't know whether to operate on the hernia or not but they're saying not at the moment, obviously hoping the problem will just re-present itself to someone else at another time. Happy Fucking Christmas.

I went for a walk on my own up to Hampstead Heath. I was obviously still quite inebriated, as I had to stop and throw up behind a tree. Maybe I'm in some sort of delayed shock. But I think I'm probably just still pissed. I went back to the house and drank more. I'll go home tomorrow, as soon as I can get a train. But for now, I'm apart from it – alone and distant, numb and cold.

## *29th December*

I went with Gareth to see Dad at the daycare centre, where he still goes once a week. After he'd asked for me on several occasions, some of the staff, along with the local authority, carried out an assessment, after which they maintained it would be too much of a risk for me to take sole care of him again. I was scared to see him, but when I got to the centre and walked up to the table where he was having lunch, he got to his feet and clung to me, with tears in his eyes. We said we would take Dad home ourselves rather than letting him go back on the bus with the rest of the mob. As we were leaving, one of the care staff mentioned that he'd told her I was his wife.

### 30th December

And so the big day has arrived. We packed some of Dad's things into a bag. Changes of clothes, shower gel, his deodorant and his favourite talc, which we placed in his old, worn, but still fully functional, leather washbag, which must have travelled with this brave and beautiful man to countries few will ever see. We had told him he was going to stay somewhere while we took a short break, but it didn't compute and to be honest I was fucking terrified about what was to come. Not least because of the attempted stabbing incident.

I remembered going to those carers' meetings with Mum and hearing how some people who'd been forced to put loved ones into care had felt absolute resentment and self-loathing. I was there now, living it. I despised what we were doing.

It was dark and cold as we walked into the centre. There was a depressed and half-hearted fake Christmas tree in the reception area, poorly decorated, melancholic and sullen. I wanted to scream.

'Checking in,' my brother said to the receptionist, dull-faced and sour (her, not him) and he gave Dad's name.

'What is this place then, kids?' Dad asked.

I didn't want to answer, but I had to. 'We're checking you in here for a bit of a rest, Dad. You know you've been through a lot and we just thought you needed some time to relax.'

'But where will you two go?' he asked, obviously worried. We didn't have time to answer. A nurse came towards us and Dad took charge immediately, standing up and striding forward with an outstretched hand.

'You know what?' he said, shaking his hand sincerely. 'In all seriousness, I think this is a very, very nice little hotel. We have been coming here for years now and I always look forward to staying with you!'

I looked to the nurse for signs of amusement, but there weren't any. Young though he was (very young), he was the embodiment of respectful professionalism. Not a smirk crossed his chops. I guess he must have heard that one before.

'It's lovely to see you again, young man!' he said, greeting Dad quietly and calmly and then taking his bags and showing him upstairs. As I went to follow, my brother held my arm.

'Let's just . . . let's . . .' Dad disappeared up the stairs and didn't look back. We went out to the car. I sat in the front seat and howled like a baby, my head in my hands. My brother stood 10 yards from the boot of the car, facing dark bushes, his shoulders shaking.

We drove with no music on and stopped in a faceless pub by the dual carriageway. In silence, we each drank two pints of piss-weak shandy in quick succession, and then we went home.

## 31st December

We haven't put up a Christmas tree, or any decorations. Guess it's too late for that now. Gareth has well and truly decided to take a break, and I'm glad. He needs it. He's flying to Africa. I guess he feels the need to return to his birthplace, perhaps for some form of reconnection and affirmation. He called me from the airport, as he was just about to board a 10-hour flight.

'What do you have planned for tonight then, kidda?'

I have been invited to a whole host of parties in London, but I don't feel like going to any of them. I want to be quiet. I want to be alone.

'Just me, Jools Holland, gin, fags and crisps.'

'Nice.' He hesitated. 'Am I . . . am I doing the right thing here? It's not right, what I'm doing.

Swanning off across the world after I've put my dad in care.'

'But this is the point. We have done this so that you can get a break. You've been dealing with him almost single-handedly since just after Mum died . . . his lowest and most difficult point. It's just not sustainable.' I tried to give my advice as impartially as possible, as if this wasn't happening to us but to someone else. 'It's not working for you and Dad can get more dedicated care this way until you feel better and we can get back on track. You need this . . . you've earned this . . . you deserve this.'

It was 6pm on the last day of the shittiest year of my life. My mum was dead, my dad was in a care home, my brother was sobbing his eyes out at 40,000 feet and I was alone, on a sofa in my family home, which contained no family and didn't feel like home. I was so far removed from reality I decided to smoke indoors. Halfway through the cigarette, I felt so ripped with guilt that I ran out to the backyard to finish it off, then I paraded through the house with a can of air freshener, just as I would have done as a young teen, disguising my sins from my parents. A rebel without a clue.

## 1st January

Happy Fucking New Year! I called the care home to check on Dad. They told me he was napping but was

OK, though he was quiet and pensive and wasn't eating much. I spent the day drifting in and out of sleep. I was hungover after drinking almost an entire bottle of gin by myself. I ran out of tonic halfway through it. Even though I'd only smoked half a cigarette indoors, the whole house stank. I had a bowl of cereal with some dubious-smelling milk. I haven't changed out of the clothes I had on yesterday, or ventured outside. I'm avoiding the New Year's well-wishers, preferring to hibernate and ignore the ringing phone instead.

## 4th January

I have decided to try to be of some use. Free of my grimy New Year's hangover, and not wanting to feel sorry for myself any longer, I have done more sorting; bagging up old bed sheets and towels to take to the tip, washing everything else, cleaning out cupboards and throwing out expired food. I defrosted the freezer, cleaned the cooker, washed all the windows and hosed down the patios. I had to feel like I was doing something. I called the care home again, but Dad didn't want to speak to me. I wanted to go and see him, but he's too far away to take the bus. My driving lessons have been so sporadic, especially since Mum died, that I don't know if I'll ever pass. I thought about asking if one of my lessons could be driving to the hospital, but then decided against it.

The same with asking someone else to drive me. I don't want to impose. I don't want to be a burden or to be indebted to anyone.

The care-home lady said Dad has been joining in and asking for newspapers and books to read. He had always been such a keen reader – and a writer. He had instilled in me his love of literature and would always buy me beautiful copies of classic titles and fully understood my reluctance to turn off my bedroom light at night and put the book down. One night, after another row with Mum over lights out, I sat in the darkness of my room in a proper sulk. I heard footsteps approaching the door and prepared myself for another round of verbal sparring. Dad stood in the doorway with a torch under his chin, pulling a ghoulish macabre face. God, he made me laugh.

'Now listen, Robs, you aren't to tell your mother about this but I used to do this as a boy. When she tells you to go to bed, put the book down and hide this quickly under your pillow. When you know you're alone again, light the torch under the duvet and you can still read your stories.'

His face was alive with mischief and the magic of a great discovery. That torch stayed under my pillow for years and saw me through many late nights. It was our secret, or so I thought. Turns out Mum knew all along, and it was parental mediation to at least get me into bed. But I knew that, really, he was on my side.

I have a lovely vision of Dad reading in his care-home room, dim, muted torchlight glowing from under stiff, starched sheets. I hope they gave him something good and not some *Mills & Boon*-type shit. He'd really hate that.

## 7th January

Dad is a fugitive – a man on the run. He has 'escaped' from his care home. Dad went out into the gardens last night after dinner and it took them ages to realise he was missing, as he made his Shawshank attempt while the staff did their shift changeover. I'm a bit angry with the care-home staff for not keeping a closer eye on him. Actually, I'm furious. We had warned them about his wandering tendencies and surely all of their charges are prone to this sort of thing?

I am staying with friends in London at the moment, or at least I was until I heard about Dad. Luckily my brother was home from Africa, but he was at the wedding of a friend. He got the call at about 11pm. Some of the staff had gone out in the car to look for him and the local police had been alerted.

Later, my brother was informed that Dad had been arrested. He'd been on a rampage while a fugitive. Apparently, two young police officers approached him on the edge of town and calmly asked him to go with them back to the care home. Dad denied any knowledge of staying there and told them to fuck off. When one of them went to put his hand on Dad he retaliated, spinning round and landing a punch right on the young policeman's jaw. With that he was wrestled to the floor, cuffed and cautioned. Dad was spitting with rage like a cornered bull, all confused and disorientated. The policemen put him in their van and took him to the station in town, where he was shut in a cell. When the care-home staff arrived he was still lashing out and making no sense. He had taken his top off and was sweating profusely, jabbering on and making wild accus-ations. Obviously, the care home had made the police aware of Dad's medical and mental situation, and they seemed to have handled him with great care and respect. The policemen who nicked him were apparently quite young, so I'm really glad they were able to demonstrate such restraint.

When the staff arrived, Dad was sedated and then released, without charge, back into their care. They wouldn't let us go to see him at the police station, which made me angry. I was worried he'd be feeling lonely and scared. He must have been terrified. I can only imagine what he thought was happening to him. Just thinking about it makes my insides curdle.

## 10th January

So, this respite care thing has not been restful in the slightest. The care home obviously hadn't met Dad's exacting standards, hence his prison break. Also, they seemed unwilling to take him back, which is kind of annoying. I didn't think such institutions got to pick and choose their patients. Anyway, he has been moved, which isn't great, as we know that any sudden and substantial change in Dad's schedule or lifestyle will cause confusion and compound his symptoms. As a bonus, he's in a home that is only about a mile and a half from the house, so I can easily walk there to see him. They have put him on painkillers and sedatives, etc., so he's not very with it. He didn't remember me today when I went to see him. I'd been warned that this would happen and although it hurt me, I knew it was better for him. He's not really here any more.

## 14th January

I went to visit Dad today. He didn't really say much, but when I went to hug him he lashed out and had to be calmed down. I don't know if he really knew who I was. What use am I to him now? I can't even visit him without causing upset. I'm stuck in my childhood house with my dad's shadow and my mum's ashes.

## 19th January

Had a cry day today, trying to keep shit together in the house, tidying and sorting, like Mum would do.

I came across a stash of old vinyl records that Dad had collected over the years. The first one I picked out was of Ella Fitzgerald and Louis Armstrong and I was transported back to Dad waltzing around the living room with me on his feet, clinging onto his waist, my little hands grabbing at his shirt and sticking my thumbs into his belt loops to stay on board. He would sing Louis Armstrong's parts and I would be Ella Fitzgerald. We would spin round and round and only stop when it got to Louis's trumpet solo, when Dad would halt on the spot and pretend to play the trumpet on his scrunched-up hands. I could smell cakes baking in the kitchen and could see Mum leaning on the doorframe watching us, smiling. I could feel his rough hands on the top of my arms as he spun me round and round again.

## 21st January

I have kept to the same routine for the past week, if you can call it that. I struggle to sleep, as I hear noises in the house all the time. I'm either on the sofa downstairs or, when my brother isn't here, in my old room upstairs. I will only go into Mum and Dad's room while it's light and I can't go into the other room Dad was staying in because it still smells of him, even though I have washed all the sheets.

When I come round from any sort of attempted slumber, I have a half-hearted shower and some tea, usually black. I haven't bought milk for ages. I then sit down and ruminate on how I ought to have handled things. What if we had known Mum was ill? Could we have arranged for better care? Should my brother and I have moved back sooner to help? Could we have pushed to get better medication for Dad? Should we have attempted to look abroad for pioneering treatment? Are Mum and Dad angry with us? Is Mum a ghost now? Does Dad miss her?

After this I get dressed (badly) and usually walk down through town, avoiding all eye contact with people. I don't want anyone to notice the mess I've become. I walk all the way to the care home. I never go in. The truth is, I'm scared of my own father, and that hurts. Sometimes I get to the door, but more often than not I sit in the car park and cry. Then I go home and try to sleep again.

## 26th January

My brother is absolutely beside himself today after going to see Dad at the home. Lately Dad has been doing much better, even though he is still pretty much mute, but a new staff member had decided to give him a haircut and also shaved off his beard. He was unrecognisable.

How can they do this? I am so angry. My brother went straight to see the home's manager and almost ripped his head off. The manager was extremely apologetic and the chap who did it was mortified. He'd assumed the beard had grown during Dad's time in care and had decided it needed taming, but he really should have asked. Dad has had his beard for as long as we have known him. It was part of his entire being. The only pictures anyone has seen of him without his beard are from his childhood. How dare they take any more of our dad away from us? You can't keep stripping away parts of a person until there is nothing left of them.

## 2nd February

I've calmed down a bit now since the beard incident, but Gareth hasn't. It was undeniably a bad judgement call from the carer, but there was no malice behind it. He really believed he was doing a good thing. I hope our reactions haven't upset him too much. I must try to ensure we speak to him when we visit this week and besides, it will grow again and he'll be back to looking like Captain Birds Eye in no time.

## 4th February

I've had some sort of breakthrough today, as I actually made it into the care home! Dad was asleep in his room so I sat outside his door and listened to him snore. That's it, that's all I did, but it feels huge. I feel closer to him now, like I've actually done things right for a change.

## 10th February

Some people are dicks. As my brother and I were driving back from the care home, where I had sat outside the door to Dad's room and read the newspapers out loud to him (I don't think he always knows what's going on as he only reacts some of the time), I called the solicitors who were dealing with our family shambles.

The firm had been recommended to Mum by somebody during one of the Alzheimer's Society's group meetings. After my dealings with this firm I couldn't help wondering why on earth anyone would recommend them. We had already been through the process of signing the documents to give us power of attorney for both our parents. I know you pay lawyers not to be emotional and to deal in hard facts, but given they were a small-town firm and we were two kids in the shit, I would have appreciated a modicum of sensitivity. They had filed the power of attorney late and missed some minor changes in the law before attempting to tell us it was our fault because we hadn't submitted our papers on time. This wasn't the case and we knew because we had logged everything and saved all our emails. The firm was just incompetent. So, after much distress, we'd asked around and enlisted the help of a family friend to act in our best interests.

I was looking forward to this phone call.

'Oh, it's you again,' was the response when I got through to the solicitor dealing with our case. Nice. 'And how can I help you today?'

The contempt was rife in her voice.

'Lovely to speak to you. I hope you're doing well?'

Silence.

'OK, then, I would like all our papers and documents back from you and your firm please,' I said, as politely as I could manage.

'What do you mean "papers and documents"?' she replied, with a thinly veiled snort.

'I mean anything you have with my family's names on them.'

'And why would you need those?' she retorted.

'Because I would like someone else to represent and help us.' I didn't sound smug or vengeful, just sad.

She didn't, though. 'So, what is it that you'd like from us, then?'

'Like I said, all the documents pertaining to the power of attorney for our father, such as his last will and testament. And anything that our mum signed that now passes to us.'

'And, like *I* said when we spoke before Christmas, I can only pass on to you any or all of your mother's documents when she's dead,' she replied haughtily.

Whoa.

'Pardon me?' I asked, stunned to the point of amusement.

'You know that. We can only pass over your mother's documents if she's dead, so . . .'

'And you do know that she IS dead? Wow, you really ought to be more up to date with your clients. Nothing's changed since 28th November. She hasn't come back to life. And just so you know, my dad's still got Alzheimer's and my brother and I are still fending off threats from the gas and electric companies because their accounts are stuck in probate.'

She tried to interrupt, but I kept going. By this point Gareth had pulled the car over to the side of the road and got me to put the call on speakerphone.

'So, as I have requested, please have all – and I do mean all – of the papers on anything to do with our family ready for me to personally collect this afternoon. If you miss anything out we will keep coming back to you and you don't want that. And as for your legal bill, well, that might get paid when their accounts get unfrozen . . . if you're lucky.'

'I'm so sorry,' she started, but then fucked up that apology, too. 'But, you know, I have been under a lot of stress lately, it's just that . . .'

'I couldn't give a shit, love. See you at three.'

I ended the call then looked at my brother. I was shaking with rage, and even my hands were trembling.

'What a twat!' he said. Then he laughed so much the car shook from mirth. We sat in the layby and almost pissed ourselves.

Needless to say, when we got to the solicitor's offices that afternoon, all our papers had been left for us with the hapless receptionist. Our solicitor was mysteriously 'unavailable'. We thanked the receptionist and ensured that she passed on to the solicitor our thanks, warmest wishes and heartfelt appreciation for going above and beyond the call of duty. The receptionist didn't catch the sarcasm in my voice (she obviously wasn't too bright because I was fairly blatant), as she looked genuinely touched. She put her hand to her chest and said, 'Ah, that's lovely, that is. I'll let her know.'

'You do that.' I smiled and left with giant paper files tucked under each arm.

## 14th February

Valentine's Day, the day of romance, but not for us. My brother and I went to see Dad again today. He was smiling and seemed happy, even though he didn't speak during our entire visit. I still don't have the guts to visit him on my own, but at least today I made it into his room to see him in person. It's been so long since I looked at him, it feels surreal, like I'm looking at him on film, perhaps. Someone else playing his character.

I watched the other patients, all of whom seemed so much older than Dad. Sometimes we saw their families, passing them with a nod and a half smile while sharing so much hurt and baggage during that brief, unspoken moment.

Today we also sat in the main hall and read to Dad. Then we both linked our arms in his and walked around the gardens. Though the ground was damp with cold winter dew, the sunshine was trying its best to smile upon the wonders of spring's gifts, a few snowdrops peeking through, some tiny buds on trees. I watched Dad's eyes to see if they picked up on anything ... to see if anyone was in there. It was as if everything had gone quiet. Senses had been dulled; there was no music.

## 18th February

You'll never guess what? I've only gone and passed my bloody driving test! I must have been the most ill-prepared test-sitter ever and almost had a crash on the way to the test centre by pulling out on someone on a dual carriageway. My instructor actually yelled.

So I got to the test centre and started out on the test route with the loveliest lady, who had a caring smile and cheery disposition. As we drove (better than I ever have, as it happens) she asked seemingly innocuous questions which I couldn't really duck.

'So, what would you usually be doing at this time of the day then? I mean, if you weren't taking a driving test?'

'Um, well, not much really,' I replied.

'Left turn here, please. Do you work?'

'I used to, not right now.'

'I see, so you're a student?' She really wasn't picking up on my evasiveness.

'Well, no, I'm caring for my father who has Alzheimer's.'

'Oh dear – oh, that's awful. Take the second exit at this roundabout, please. My mother had that, too, it's such a wretched disease.'

I carried on as per her instructions, and bizarrely the chat eased the test tension.

'He has been taken into care so that's eased things a bit,' I continued.

'I doubt it's eased it much; you still have the worry, you poor thing. You're so young! Please pull up on this side of the road after the big truck, wherever is safe.'

I then performed a near-perfect parallel park, and I always fuck those up. I pulled off again.

'And how is your mother coping? Take the right turn onto the main road here please.'

'Mum passed away just before Christmas . . .'

'Flipping heck! You have been through it, haven't you? Take the second left after the school and back into the test centre where I would like you to reverse into a space of your choice.'

Again, the manoeuvre was perfection; she thanked

me and asked me to switch off the engine. Without feeling or melancholy I awaited the sentence starting with, 'On this occasion I regret to tell you that . . .'

Except those weren't the words that came.

'Robyn, I am thrilled to tell you that you have passed . . .' and before she could continue I burst into tears over the steering wheel of a Citroen Saxo.

'Oh now, my dear, you've done so well,' she said sympathetically, as she patted my shoulder.

We got out of the car and walked back to the reception area where my instructor was waiting. He stood up with a 'never mind, you can have more lessons with me' face and I told him I'd passed.

'What?! Really?! Are you sure that's what she said?' he replied, more genuinely concerned than surprised. He drove me home and I thanked him for all his work. He remained grim-faced.

G was waiting by the front door as I gleefully danced up the path shaking my pass papers.

'I knew you would do it, kidda!' he said, enveloping me in a big hug.

The next day he went to see Dad and told him the news. Dad was mute and slouched on a sofa. G took his hand and said, 'Hey, Dad, you know what happened yesterday? Robyn passed her driving test!'

I don't know if this is G embellishing for the sake of a story, but it may well be true. Dad let out a snuffled grunt and his hand spasmed tightly round Gareth's.

Cheeky git.

## *1st* **March**

Happy St David's Day. Or, if you speak Welsh, Dydd Gwyl Dewi Hapus. I don't, apart from that. My brother and I went to see Dad again today. He is much better. He apparently spoke this morning and had breakfast. I like to allow myself (only momentarily) to think this means something, that he will continue to improve as his brain comes back to him and he returns to the man he was . . . our dad. It's a selfish and wretched thought that makes me smile for the very, very brief second I allow myself to believe. We took in some parts of *The Sunday Times* to read aloud to him. I did the business section and my brother tackled the sport. I took a walk in the gardens of the home and picked some daffodils. I asked the nurses for a vase or tumbler to put them in and placed them on the windowsill of Dad's room, where we sat for hours in the pale, spring afternoon sunshine.

My brother asked the wardens if he could give Dad a beer to toast St David's Day with. They kind of agreed, in a way that intimated it wasn't really agreeable, but the poor man is dying and if the only thing we can do for him is to give him a decent drink then, yes, of course we could.

G had sourced a rare Kenyan lager that Dad loved. We have pictures of G stealing Dad's beer in Africa, his little toddler potbelly is hanging over his terry towelling shorts as he sneaks up behind Dad, who is deep in conversation, to take a slurp.

We quietly cracked open three bottles in his room and swigged away. The faint smile on Dad's face was beautiful, and I hope that in some way he was transported back to those times in Africa. Whether his memories were real or invented, I wished for those sips to take him somewhere better than this.

### 8th March

I've been in London staying with a friend for a few days. I've done very little apart from walk around the city. It was nice weather and I felt alone and free. I managed a smile, too, but then I thought of Mum and Dad and the guilt I felt for having experienced a small moment of happiness was worse than having never smiled at all.

### 10th March

Dad has pneumonia. He's now on a drip and my brother says he doesn't look like our dad any more. He's on bed rest and his carers are cautious about visitors, so we have been told not to see him for a few days. I came home from London as soon as I heard, and did my old trick of walking to the home and sitting in reception for a while, talking to the nurses as they walked around. I asked about Dad, chatted to some of the other patients and generally tried to offer my help. One very elderly and frail lady came to sit with me. She seemed compos mentis and told me that her daughter was coming to collect her. She had her coat over her arm and was clutching a handbag, from which she kept removing tissues. She offered me one and I accepted it, as it seemed rude to decline the offer. We must have sat for over an hour talking about nothing and everything. Then one of the nurses came out and called the lady in for lunch.

'But my daughter,' the elderly lady said. 'How will she know where I am? I don't want her to miss me or to think I have left without her.'

'It's all right, if she arrives we will come and get you,' the nurse replied kindly, with a wink.

'Well, I'll be here for a little while,' I said. 'So if she arrives I can let someone know.'

The lady thanked me and then scowled at the nurse.

On her return from ushering patients into the dining room, the nurse stopped by me. 'She sits there most days and waits for her daughter,' she explained. 'But she lives in America and hasn't been here for almost a year now. We try not to correct her. Sometimes it's better for them to have hope.'

Isn't that true of us all?

# *18th March*

Visiting Dad today was the most upsetting experience of my life. This is his first day out of his pneumonia-induced solitary confinement. I am shocked, distressed and disturbed. This vision of him will haunt me for ever. It felt as if someone was playing a strange and horrible joke on me, and that at any moment Dad would snap out of it and let us know that he was playing around. It was too extreme to believe, too much of a change. His face was so gaunt. He didn't have his teeth in, and, apparently, he no longer uses them. He has been having severe trouble swallowing food and drink, so the nurses have to be careful when feeding him, mushing up all his food for him. His eyes were vacant and he looked as if some horrible force had sucked his soul right out of him. He can't walk properly and kind of shuffles around, even then with assistance. He has lost so much weight and resembles a frail skeleton that no longer wants to be of this world.

My brother came with me to the care home, and when we arrived the staff said Dad was on the sofa. One of the nurses went over to get him up and I was so taken aback when they sat him up that I burst into tears. His mouth just kind of hung open and his eyes were no longer the sparkling blue they used to be; they were now dark, deep, expressionless holes. They might as well have bored right through his head and out the other side – there is nothing there any more. My lovely dad is a zombie, his wonderful brain hollow and still. Sometimes I think of him as an abandoned building, like those pictures of derelict hospitals you see, where all the apparatus is still in situ but now gathering dust. Quiet and still, haunted and eerie, just the outer walls still standing.

A nurse sat Dad up and put her arm across his shoulder.

'Look, look who's here to see you,' she said. 'It's your son and daughter.'

Dad looked in our direction, but his eyes didn't focus. He just let out a dull, pained moan. At that point I rushed out of the main building. I sat out in the reception and cried until I realised that someone was sitting next to me with their hand on mine.

'I know it's hard, love. You haven't seen him properly in almost two weeks and it's not long since you lost your mam. It's never easy but you must know that he is comfortable. It don't seem like it, I know, but he is here and we are giving him all the love and care we can.'

Her voice was soft and warm. She sounded like a teacher I had at infant school, the sing-song cadence of her accent like a slow rocking action that was easy to lose yourself to.

'I just lost my dad to Alzheimer's seven weeks ago,' she continued. 'It's hard but I do believe he knows . . . . he knows that you're here . . . he knows that you love him.'

She was a lovely nurse, very round with a harsh, dark bob with striking streaks of red through it, and many bad tattoos. She reminded me of a character from *The Twits* by Roald Dahl, about whom the author says, 'But if you have good thoughts they will shine out of your face like sunbeams and you will always look lovely.'

'Do you know what I find helps, my love?' she replied before I could answer. 'Cider. I loves cider, I do. I got some cans in my fridge at home. And some leftover Chinese, so I'll have that, too, when I get back after my shift.'

She zoned out as she imagined looking into her kitchen fridge. 'I hope you get some cider.' She smiled.

It was the most bizarre consolation ever, and totally heartfelt. I actually hate cider, but she made me smile.

After the pep talk, she gave me some tissues and left. I stood up and could see my dad and brother through the glass. Dad was walking around while Gareth supported him, holding his arm. I felt sick. Dad scared me. He looked like a corpse already . . . I didn't want to be frightened of my own dad. He looked so helpless and I also felt so, so sorry for him. I should have been there to look after him more. I was upset that I couldn't provide him with the care and love that he needed and deserved. I felt as if I had abandoned him in the care home and I will never ever shake the guilt that hangs around my neck like a heavy chain and causes my shoulders to ache. This will burden me for all time.

Another nurse came out to see me, asking if I would go back in with her. I took some convincing, and I thought it was a little unfair as I was so obviously uncomfortable, but I went back in nonetheless. G was standing with Dad, feeding him a cup of tea. When he saw me he gently lowered the cup from Dad's mouth.

'Look, Dad. Look who's here.'

Dad looked in my direction, but our eyes never met. I reached my hand out and touched his. It was cold, damp and lifeless.

'Hiya, Dad, it's just me . . . how are you? You all right?'

And that was it. I was lost for words and just couldn't think of what to say next. What do you say to someone who can't hear you? That's a stupid question. Just then it came to me. I knew exactly what to say.

'I just wanted to stop by and tell you something, Dad,' I said softly. 'I love you very, very much, I do. I love you, Dad.'

Dad gripped my hand tight, just like he used to when I was little and he thought I might run away. I felt like I could run away right then, run as far as I could possibly go. I just didn't want to deal with it. If I could go away somewhere warm, near a beach, I could pretend this wasn't happening and be happy. If I ran, I would have no problems. He let out another moan from his toothless, black hole of a mouth.

'I'm sorry, I can't . . . I think I need some air.'

I ran to the toilet, threw up and sat and cried until the nurse who'd persuaded me to see him again came knocking on the door. She went to get my brother. We walked out to the car park and I cried all the way home. Later, he took me to the pub for lunch. It felt like all those times Dad had taken us to the pub for food as kids. I didn't feel much older now. We both ordered burgers. My brother had a Coke; I had half a cider.

## 23rd March

Today, following a rainstorm, I walked down to see Dad. The streets smelled of rain and it made me think of walking home from school, mud splattering up the backs of my legs and damp uniform clinging to my skin. I like the way the streets smell after rain, cleaner, purged, like a new start. The sun was breaking out and brightening the inky blue of the sky, and there was a big, beautiful rainbow. From the top of the hill it looked as if it ended just over the care home, except the closer I got, the further it moved away. It was teasing and taunting me, as if it didn't want to commit.

When I arrived, Dad looked as if he had been crying. He was sitting on the sofa, his head hung low. He didn't seem to notice me as I sidled up to him and slid my hand into his. I did nothing for an hour and a half. I just sat with my head on his shoulder and my hand in his hand. I could feel his breath on my hair and could almost hear his heart beating through his pullover.

When the staff indicated it was time for me to leave, I couldn't even say goodbye, but I like to think I felt Dad squeeze my hand.

## 2nd April

Dad has contracted pneumonia again. I don't see how this can happen to a person who doesn't go outdoors. I've always associated the infection with folk who climb Everest or something. But anyway, he is on a drip and off his food again. Gareth says he is so unrecognisable now that I might find seeing him too upsetting. So when we went to visit him today, I stayed by the door, reading out loud from the newspapers and back copies of *Private Eye*. The understanding wardens and nurses brought me cups of tea, blankets and cushions. I slept and dribbled by the door for hours until it was time to go home and shower, eat, rest and repeat.

Even though I didn't have the courage to go into Dad's room, I hope he knew I was there.

## 4th April

Another day, another issue. Dad is having trouble swallowing and eating, they have to mash his food

up most of the time now and feed him like a baby.
We had a meeting with the home manager who
suggested that at some point they may need to feed
him subcutaneously. We asked for clarification on
what that was and was told it involved feeding him
through a tube into his stomach. It's a last resort and
is reserved for end-of-life care. Fuck that. I don't
want them to cut my dad up just to prolong this hell.
There is no way he would want that to happen.

## 8th April

I'm still trying to find humour in this mire of shit.
It got to 'closing time' at the home today and my
brother came to wake me. I was sleeping like a
tramp under a pile of blankets by Dad's door. The
care-home manager took pity on us and offered my
brother and me beds.

'You know you are both welcome to stay here,'
he said. 'It's not conventional but we do have
some spare beds this month. I recognise that times
are tough for you both and I'd like to offer you
something.'

He was so kind and genuine, but I had to bite
my lip to stop myself from laughing. I was too
squeamish to sit with my own father, so I certainly
couldn't comprehend sleeping in a bed in the room
next door. It was funny, but also so sweet of him.
We declined and went home to eat beans on toast.

My brother suggested watching a movie, to take our minds off everything, but in the end we both fell asleep on the sofa with all the lights on and our plates on our laps.

## 10th April

Day by day I have inched closer into Dad's room. Today I made it to the foot of his bed, but I was still too scared to look him in the face. I don't want to see him if he doesn't look like my dad any more. I don't want that to stay with me. He is already being taken from us, and I don't want the good memories of our 'last times' to be stolen, too.

My brother sat in a chair and I positioned myself on the floor, touching his hand and stroking his old fingers. He barely made a move, barely made a sound. We found an odd sort of peace.

The staff ambled silently round us, smiling softly but not making eye contact. They knew what was coming.

## 13th April

Today we spent an hour or so with Dad after his evening meal before going off to have some dinner ourselves. It wasn't that the food there triggered any sort of appetite, but we realised that neither of us could remember when we had last eaten. The phone call came as soon as we had arrived back at the house and settled on the sofa.

'Hello, it's the care home here. It's about your dad,' said the meek-voiced caller. 'He's, um, he's very, um . . .'

Dead, I was thinking. Just tell me he's dead.

'He's very near. I was just thinking you might like to come back, if you want to. It's up to you, kids, but we just wanted to let you know.'

I hung up the phone and turned to look at my brother, who had his mouth open, even though it was half-full of chocolate biscuit. It was pretty gross, but it wasn't the most pressing issue. He looked frozen in time. I thought about how we'd been together in this room when the night nurse had come down to tell us Mum was breathing her last. It was only four months ago, which felt like a lifetime, and yet no time at all. For some reason, I remembered how she'd woken Gareth up by wiggling his big toe, which was sticking out of the tiny tartan blanket he'd used to cover himself. I almost laughed at the memory, then half cried. Then I just said, 'Shut your mouth, I can see your Twix.'

'Is he dead?' Gareth managed to sputter through the biscuit.

'Not quite. The nurse said we might want to go back.'

My brother was still holding his car keys. As if on autopilot, he shovelled the rest of the Twix into his mouth and made for the front door.

When we got back to the care home there were only a few cars about. It was eerily quiet; a still night with not even moonlight or stars or sound – just blackness. The lights were dim in the home, weak glows emitted from distant rooms and the small, pink-clad shape of the nurse, clutching tissues in her hand, came closer to us.

She took my brother in one hand and me in the other. I got the one with the damp tissue in it. It remained clamped between us as she took us to the chairs outside Dad's room. She led us like a teacher would lead very young children.

'I'm so sorry for your loss,' she said. 'He passed just a few minutes ago. It was very peaceful.'

All I could think about was how we should never have left the hospital and also that I didn't get a Twix.

The question was posed again. 'Would you like to see him?'

I wanted to snap back: 'No, I didn't want to see my dead mother and I don't want to see my dead father!'

Luckily, G stepped in, as he always does, kindly and delicately handling everything with his clumsy grace.

'Yes, I would, but I think my sister would prefer not to.'

The nurse nodded in appreciation and said kindly, 'Of course, each to their own.'

My brother was the man; he needed to manage, to deal, to cope. I was the baby and I needed to be protected – a 26-year-old baby. An orphan. Are we too old to be orphans? That's what we are now. Orphans.

'Well, then, I shall give you all the time and space you need, while you and I' – she turned to me – 'make some tea.'

The nurse led me away by the hand and I didn't even feel my feet move. Even though lots of things were going on in my head, I wondered what other people would see. Did I look shocked? Did I look like someone who had just lost someone? My brother didn't look any different to me. Did I to him?

It was one of the worst cups of tea I have ever had in my life. Piss weak. But I got a biscuit, one of the circular shortbread ones covered in sugar. The nurse informed me it would be good for the shock, so I must have looked shocked then.

'We haven't had a death here in a very long time,' she informed me with wide eyes.

Good chat, I thought.

'I'm sorry,' I said.

'My dear, whatever for? We are here to look after and care for people, to hopefully make them better, but to make them comfortable if we can't. This is our job.'

She sounded calm, but proud, especially when she said the last bit.

My brother came in.

'I've made you a cup of tea,' the nurse proclaimed, 'with extra sugar for the shock.'

I managed a sly smile when we locked eyes, then I started to wail. My brother held me close and I felt his tears and dribble in my hair. He drank his tea like a good little boy . . . like a boy who wouldn't want to insult someone for their kindly deed.

I don't recall getting home.

## 14th April

It took me a few seconds this morning to remember that I had no parents. I'd slept in my clothes, quite well it would seem. Odd. My brother was downstairs watching *Takeshi's Castle* again.

'All right?'

'Yeah,' he said. 'You all right?'

'Yeah, I guess so.'

'We've got to go and see the funeral directors again. Fun.' His face settled in firm-jawed misery.

'Well, technically we don't have to do anything now.'

'How do you mean?' He frowned.

'Well, we have no grown-ups to tell us off.' I grinned.

'You're a prick. I'm having a shower,' he replied, walking off.

'Did you sleep?' I called after him.

He stopped, his back still to me. 'I don't even know.'

After we had pulled into the funeral parlour car park, we waited for a song on the radio to stop playing before we got out of the car. It was 'Round Here' by Counting Crows. I used to love that song, and whenever I hear it I think of being at school in the 90s and wearing Dr. Martens.

The funeral director was shocked to see us again. He offered tea, which I accepted and my brother refused. He's had enough of death and he's had enough of tea.

'It saddens me to see you two here so soon, it really does,' the funeral director said. 'But if we can take any solace in this it is that your mother and father are together again. Now, I know you two aren't particularly religious, and to tell you a little secret neither am I, but I really do believe that.'

In a way, I did, too. Even if what he was saying was just fancy bullshit to get me through the day, it worked and I grasped at it wholeheartedly.

We chose daffodils for the funeral, as they seemed appropriate for a Welshman, even though Dad's Welshness wasn't something bestowed upon him by birth but imposed upon him by war.

We decided to send him off in his naval uniform. We used to joke and call Dad Uncle Albert after the character in *Only Fools and Horses*, but in reality he hadn't fought in any war. As a fully trained engineer, he'd formed part of the Merchant Navy. When he and Mum met in Chelsea in the late 60s, he was constantly being called away to the ship. When they married she went with him, and they sailed around the world several times over before settling in Kenya. Anyway, as he'd lost some timber through being ill we thought he'd fit nicely back into his uniform. It felt like the right thing to do. He was a proud man.

We chose music by John Barry, just as we had for Mum's funeral, and we went with a song called 'Flying Over Africa'. I hoped that when we played it at the funeral that's where Mum and Dad would be: together in his old twin-seated prop plane in the mid-70s. Dad holding Mum's hand, both of them golden and glowing as they glided in the blue sky over their beloved Kenyan landscape. Dad would be wearing his old aviator glasses and Mum would be looking down, pointing excitedly at herds of elephants. They would be in love and together and nothing would be able to touch them.

## 19th April

The same people and family again – the same cars, the same drill. Honestly, it was like *Groundhog Day*. But where I feel I kept my shit together at Mum's funeral, today I couldn't cope at all. I'd managed to speak at Mum's ceremony and gave a warm eulogy, but at Dad's I couldn't stop crying. I did stand up to read a poem with a very wobbly voice, but I only just made it through. We managed to have one laugh, though. It was only my brother and me at the front pew, as everyone else stayed back a bit. The vicar, the same vicar who knew our family and had presided over Mum's funeral, spoke wonderfully, again. She mentioned some of Dad's global, work-related achievements; how he'd helped to build power stations all over the world, including in some remote and dangerous places. In particular, she pointed out his efforts to stop the River Nile flowing for 30 minutes while he checked the dam. It was all very impressive.

'And when his children told me of these wondrous moments, I wasn't shocked,' she said. 'He was an amazing man, but I do wish I had asked him about these things in more detail.'

As she spoke, she moved closer to the coffin before placing a hand on it, leaning on it quite heavily and adding, 'But I guess it's too late now.' As a final flourish, she looked longingly at the box.

At that point my brother and I locked eyes and dissolved into the most childish burst of hysterics. It was all just so overdramatic. We share the same odd sense of humour and we had to hold each other up while stifling our sniggering.

After the funeral, a close friend approached us.

'God, I felt for you so much, especially at the church,' they said. 'I could see your shoulders shaking and I could feel your pain.'

I guess it wasn't quite the right moment to share the joke.

The wake was at least a little less desperate than Mum's. I didn't have to watch out for Dad trying to start a conga, but at the same time it just felt so final, so bleak. And I was totally exhausted. My brother had managed to source a few cases of the Kenyan lager that Dad had loved so much and he opened them at the bar and encouraged everyone to take one for the toast. The speech he gave was wonderful and seemed full of hope and gratitude, but knowing my brother it was for the people present, so they wouldn't feel too sorry for us or worry about us too much. That's his way. He makes people feel at ease and never shows his problems. We are like that as a family. I could see our parents' actions echo and ripple right through us both. Here we stood, both so private in our grief, solemn and composed: no cracks, no signs – a stiff upper lip.

From the wake back to the house it was just the two of us in the limousine. It was such a big car for two . . . two orphans. I felt very small and I'm sure he did, too. Our legs seemed to stick straight out over the edge of the seats, our feet not reaching the floor. The black leather interior was dampening all sound and drowning all feeling. Our hands met in the middle of the back seat. Our fingertips were touching just enough to let each other know we were there. We looked out of our respective windows at our town crawling by, all grey and sad. We were alone – but together alone.

## 20th April

We returned to the care home today. We wanted to give the staff something to thank them for looking after Dad, so we took in some big bunches of flowers, two large tins of chocolates and a thank-you card. Mum always taught us to write thank-you cards. The nurses and staff seemed shocked. I hope that other people buy them flowers and treats. I just wanted to acknowledge the fact that we were aware Dad had been a bit of a handful at times. The manager, in particular, seemed very appreciative but a bit hesitant, like he was hiding something. He had a small bag containing some of Dad's things, including his pyjamas and some books. We didn't really want them but it seemed churlish to tell the manager to throw them in the bin. He seemed reluctant to hand them over.

'There's something else,' he began. 'Your father asked us a lot for pencils and notepaper.'

This wasn't a surprise, as he loved to write.

'He asked us to post some letters for him. Now, I hope you don't think we were being sneaky or anything, and I guess we really ought to have mentioned this earlier, but, well, we have kept everything as it was. You might like to take a look.'

I sat down at his office desk, my brother at my shoulder, and carefully took out some folded notepapers, which had been prudently enclosed within a slim paperclip. There were about six or seven hand-written letters from Dad, written to his best man, with whom he had lived in London when he and Mum started dating. Dad was telling him how he had been captured and was being held against his will. He had tried to describe his surroundings and location so that he might be found and rescued, but the details had all become jumbled and nonsensical. In many cases the letters tailed off into childish squiggly lines and doodles. He had folded each notelet up and, in the absence of an envelope, written his best man's name on the front followed by 'London, SW3'.

It was too sad for words, especially because the man in question had been killed in an awful accident in South Africa only a few years after Mum and Dad got married.

### 21st April

Another urn of ashes. Dad seemed lighter than Mum. We brought him home and put him on the bookcase alongside his wife. They are now side by side, looking out of the window over the town. We drove to the supermarket to pick up some food for tea, and when we came in we both shouted up to our parents in their bedroom.

'Hi, Mum, hi, Dad!' we called and then smiled. We set about making some dinner and messing about in the kitchen, arguing grotesquely about who would get what from the house. My brother wanted some of their beautiful African sculptures and pictures, while I wanted the Papua New Guinea butterflies in cases. Although they were beautifully macabre, they reminded me of my childhood and the few years we had spent there.

We got onto the subject of Dad's old wooden captain's chair. It was cracked and ancient and we had sat in it for so many family photographs, perched on our parents' laps, wearing the smart clothes we'd been forced into, and coerced into smiling. Right now it was up in their room, by the window, where we sat to talk to their ashes.

'So, technically, I should get it as I'm the oldest and that's what happens. The firstborn gets first pick.'

'Oh, is that how it goes? That's the law, is it?' I said, laughing.

'Yeah, and also, I'm the son and heir, you're the daughter and spare.'

'For fuck's sake, you're going to play the cock card, are you? Really? Hilarious.'

He moved towards me, put me in a head lock and did that annoying thing he used to do when we were kids, whereby he viciously rubbed his knuckles over my head until I yelled for mercy.

'Ah, no, stop . . . stop. Mum! Dad! Tell hiiiiiiimmmmm!' I screamed between spits of giggles.

Then all of a sudden we heard a huge thump from upstairs. It sounded like it was coming from their bedroom.

We ripped ourselves apart instantly and stood up straight. My brother whimpered like a puppy and I went to go for the back door.

'What the fuck?! Go up there and see what that was,' he said.

'Nope, you're the oldest. You go, big brother.'
'Come with me.' He looked like he did as a young boy, when we used to scare each other with ghost stories.

'Fuck off.'

'They're mad. They're mad at us for rowing.'

'They're mad at you for being a dick,' I said. Then I yelled into the silence. 'Give us a sign if you think he ought to get the captain's chair.'

My brother ran for the back door, shoving me out of the way so hard I fell over onto the kitchen floor. I was laughing and powerless.

When we recovered we ate dinner on our laps in front of the telly. We both slept on the sofas that night.

### 30th April

Sometimes I like our small town and sometimes I hate it. Today I missed London's anonymity. My brother has gone to stay with some friends on the south coast. I've stayed in the house on my own and haven't left it for four days. I haven't washed and I haven't changed my clothes, and it was only an absolute necessity that drove me into the real world once more. I had run out of food and toilet paper. If I hadn't I wouldn't have ventured outside the safe cocoon of the house. I fumbled my greasy hair into a ponytail and wiped away the remainder of the eye make-up I had put on many days ago but then failed to remove.

On walking down the steep hill, I became acutely aware of how badly I smelled. And I wasn't wearing any underwear, I can't remember when I last wore underwear. In the supermarket I became paranoid that people were looking at me and seeing only a horrid, stinky mess. I was so ashamed of myself. Then an old friend of my mum approached me in the dairy aisle. Although she was speaking directly to me, I couldn't really hear what she was saying. It was as if the volume wasn't turned right the way up. I don't recall saying goodbye to her, but I do remember leaving my entire basket of groceries on the floor in the middle of the shop and walking out without anything. I cried all the way up the hill, vicious salty tears carving chasms down my face, neck and under my smelly sweatshirt. When I got to the house some kind person had left a gift on the doorstep. Along with another bunch of flowers and a hoard of sympathy cards, there was a large earthenware dish of lasagne. It was still warm and it was so, so welcome. I took it into the house with the rest of the things and suddenly, a savage hunger tore through my body – like I was just waking up or coming round. I ate some of the lasagne, made myself a cup of tea and ran a hot bath with lots of bubbles. After that I watched some evening news and ate more of the lasagne. I was clean, warm and fed. Whoever made that lasagne knew it was exactly what I didn't know I needed. You brought me back to life, sweet friend.

## 12th May

As we have so many weird and wonderful artefacts in our house, my brother and I decided to enlist the help of an expert to discuss whether anything might be of value. It's not like we are seeking money from misery, far from it. But, you know, we are orphans now and we feel like we're due some luck. Plus, I'm quite broke, having not had an income for eight months, with the exception of my carer's allowance, which I'm now going to have to cancel.

So I called some chap from a rather well-known auction house and, after describing some of the items we had been bequeathed, he said he'd pop round for a look. For the occasion I bought in biscuits. Good ones, none of that value stuff from Tesco.

Sadly, the bloke was a prick. I knew it as soon as I saw him pull up at the house, get out of his car and straighten his bow tie. I greeted him at the door and put on my best phone voice. I didn't let my Valley's lilt slip out once. The man had a limp handshake, which compounded my first impression. Mum used to warn me about people with limp handshakes – don't trust them.

So anyway, he skulked around the house, peering down through the small-lensed spectacles that were balanced at the end of his long, ruddy nose. He walked with his hands clasped behind his back, a little bit like Dad used to, but that is where the nice comparisons end. I showed him antique after antique. He declared an original Edison phonograph 'passé', a giant, late nineteenth-century American wall clock 'more than ten a penny' and questioned why anyone would want a set of rare Papua New Guinean tribal spears. I could certainly think of a few reasons . . .

I offered him tea and set the biscuits on the table (1960s original McIntosh – deemed 'pedestrian') and brought some old books over for inspection. His interest piqued.

'Well, I say,' he began, sliding his specs further up his nose and straightening his back. 'If this book is one of the first limited editions it might be worth thousands!'

It was my dad's copy of *The Source of the Nile* by John Hanning Speke. He loved that book. I pictured him reading it while the antiques chump plucked a reference book out of his briefcase, donned some white cotton gloves and fingered the pages with care. I left him for a moment while I re-boiled the kettle, returning to a big sigh.

'Well, sadly, this *isn't* the first edition as I had hoped, it's from a later print run. It's probably only worth a few hundred.'

This was more than I had right now, so I was pretty impressed.

'Nothing of value then?' I enquired. I was tiring of this man's shitty attitude, how he'd looked my house up and down with disdain because we didn't live in some big mansion.

'*Au contraire*,' the man sneered. 'In your father's latter stages of dementia, he seems to have taken to using money as a bookmark.'

With that he flicked up a crisp and pristine £20 note. Pressing it between his first and second fingers, he held it aloft and looked over his glasses at me.

'Ha! The dopey old bastard!' I exclaimed, snatching the note swiftly from his slimy grasp.

While smiling at it, mesmerised and soothed somehow, Mr Sneery got out of the chair, straightened his bow tie once more and headed for the door. I trailed half-heartedly after him, £20 note still in hand, gazing at it and thinking that its place may have marked the last words my dad had ever read. When we got to the door, the man turned to bid me farewell and held out his hand with such indifference that I didn't even bother to shake it or meet his gaze. I just closed the door in his face and clutched the note to my chest with a smile.

Fortunately, he hadn't even touched the biscuits.

# 4th June

The house has sold! It's all happening so quickly. Someone has put in a reasonable offer in cash and they want to move in as soon as possible. My brother is making enquiries about storage and house clearance. I am fretting over whether we are doing the right thing. Neither of us wants to sell up, but what are we keeping the house for? Is it time to move on, or is it too soon? Are we abandoning our parents by selling the house? Should we continue to stand by our family, even though we don't really have one any more? Am I supposed to go back to London now, as if nothing's happened? As if I had just taken a brief sabbatical of shite? Are we both supposed to return to our old lives as they were . . . as we were? Or do we stay here and mourn and wallow? How much time is too much time? I have so many questions that no one can answer.

But there is one thing we both know we need to do. It is something that neither of us have so far broached, so it has been unspoken.

My brother came downstairs with an urn under each arm. 'Come on, sis, it's time,' he said.

We both knew where we were heading. My brother drove to the top of the mountains overlooking town. From the top you can see for miles and miles, right over the Somerset coast. Sometimes we used to skip school up here. It is especially beautiful on a clear June day, with the mild sunshine and cheeky winds. Mum and Dad used to love walking up here. I thought this would give them a good view over everything for ever more. It's a good resting place.

My brother took Mum while I took Dad. Walking up to the highest point, breathlessly leaning into the wind and negotiating the mounds of bracken and rocky patches, we found our perfect point and unscrewed the lids.

'Ready?' he asked.

'Yup, ready.'

And with that we whirled round and round, spinning the ashes into the wind and clouds, and up into the sky. They danced on the mild breeze, like swarms of migrating birds that move as part of something far bigger than themselves. We shook out the last of the ashes and watched the wind whip them in and out of the patchy sunshine. We followed them as they drifted and sailed and soared from something into nothing . . . into the ether and everywhere.

## 18th June

So today I left the house. It's a house of memories, both sad and happy. I'd held mixed emotions about this house, my house, but not any more. It was our time to move on now, and hopefully time for a new family to begin to build their happy memories.

I read somewhere that we never really own a house, we are merely caretakers or custodians, so I hope the terrace has found some loving new incumbents; it deserves joy, as it has given us so much over the years – excluding the last few months. But those sad days shouldn't tarnish an otherwise beautiful life. This is just what people have to do, isn't it? At some point, everyone has to say goodbye to their parents. Like they say, dying is just a part of life.

I posted the keys back through the letterbox, zipped up my leather jacket, slung my large bag with the last of my possessions from Wales over my shoulder and started walking. Most of my stuff is now in storage. For how long, who knows? I walked all the way down the steep hill, the big view from the top fading away. I got on the bus and watched the rows of tiny houses as I passed. Those damp Valley towns, with their faintest glimmer and glitter of sunshine. Everything seemed small again.

I boarded the little train at the station, then changed trains when I reached town, onto the big Paddington one. I didn't sleep. Instead, I intently watched the fields and farms speed by, the villages and towns growing bigger as we neared the city, the sky getting brighter. I pulled into London as pale summer sunshine peeked through the smog and the smoke, the hustle and the bustle, the people and the noise, the comfort and the anonymity. I thought about how no one walking past me had any idea of what I'd just been through, what I am going through, but then again, I could say the same for them. How do you ever really know another person's story? I walked out onto the main street, hailed the 27 bus and rode it all the way back to Camden. I had no idea what lay ahead today, tonight or tomorrow. I felt sad but buoyed, hollow but hardened, broken but sharp, sad but hopeful.

Deep down, I had a feeling that everything would just . . .

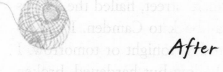

# After

## November 2016

Dear Mum and Dad,

G came down for the weekend. They left last night, him, his girlfriend and their son. He's really growing up fast, isn't he? Six years old already! But I know you're watching, I know you know. They stayed with us here in our little flat and we walked in Richmond Park, as we always do. I feel you both with me when I walk there, and I know you would have loved to stay with us, my husband and me and our doggy.

Although we speak every day I don't know if you know how much I think of you, especially as it's almost ten years since you both moved on. It's weird to think that you haven't aged, but that we have. I don't dream about you being ill. In my dreams, you look the same, you are well, happy and fit. Back in your prime. They are nice dreams now.

It hasn't been easy for us without you, especially early on. I know you watched when I screwed a lot of things up. You watched when I continually fell down and couldn't get back up. You watched as I refused to acknowledge that I needed help. You watched when I finally admitted that I had to get my shit back together. It must have been painful to see, especially as you couldn't help me. And I needed your help so badly. The only people that could fix me were the only people who weren't able to. I am sorry if I disappointed you. I hope that you are proud of me now; I know you were proud of me before you went.

And I know you'll be proud of G. He's a terrific dad. It's sad that you never got to be grandparents, you'd have been wonderful. G says all the time that as he watches his son grow up, he understands so much more about his relationship with you. I, for one, know that I was a naughty little shit!

Both G and I knew you were there when I got married to Andy nearly six years ago. Obviously Gareth gave me away, in the same church where we said goodbye to you both. G cried a lot that day. All your friends came, too, and all the family. I feel as if you sent Andy to me and I'm gutted you never got to meet him, but as G said in his father-of-the-bride speech that day, 'Mum and Dad may not have met you but you were known to them'.

When Andy and I moved into our first place together in London, a few years after you both went, I got some of our beautiful things from storage and went about feathering our nest together, combining me and him with a sense of you two. I unpacked a box while we ate fish and chips and drank champagne, and pulled out a little card I had made for you, Mum, when you were ill when I was about 10 years old (the only time you were ever ill before you died – great sick record, Mum!). In my childish biro scribbles, there was a stick person in a bed surrounded by flowers. Inside, I'd written I had a new boyfriend called Andrew and that I think I loved him enough to marry him, my infantile handwriting carefully rendered on prepared pencilled lines. And so it was that my junior-school boyfriend came back into my life some 20 years later to sweep me off my feet and turn my life around. Thank you, Mum, for making that happen! His parents are great, too; they love me and look after me like I was their own but, you know, with less ribbing and banter.

The last few months have been challenging in a different sort of way. After going back into fashion and even setting up my own company, it is definitely time for change. I have you both to thank for my sense of adventure, for my lack of fear about dropping a successful career to chase something potentially futile – writing this book.

I revisited my old diary the other month, the one I kept all those years ago, when you got ill. Opening that Pandora's box of feelings was extremely painful but also therapeutic. It made me feel closer to you but at the same time what happened felt distant, like a nightmare I couldn't quite remember the details of. I took a self-critical look at things I could have and should have done differently, but I'm always like that. As you always used to say, Mum, there's always someone out there worse off than you, and despite losing you both, I agree, I was lucky to have had you at all. It also made me feel sanguine somehow – if I can get through that then there's plenty more I can accomplish.

I wondered about self-publishing my diary, purely for cathartic reasons, to exhume some old ghosts. Then, on your birthday, Dad, I spoke with an agent who wanted to publish it properly! She said you sounded great (I told her you were), and in the few short weeks since then we have chosen a publisher to work with. Oddly enough, both my agent and my publisher are Welsh. I'm not sure if their lineage directly affected my decision, but I felt that they really 'got' us and that your story – our story – would be safe in their hands.

So that leads us to now. I am finishing editing bits and pieces, choosing cover designs, dotting Is and crossing Ts, sitting at my little antique bureau that Andy bought me, under the warm glow of an old banker's lamp in our kitchen, dog snoring softly at my feet.

I'm not sure how this book will be received, or what people will think. After you got ill, Dad, and I had just moved back, I remember often feeling embarrassed by Alzheimer's and what the disease did to you. I still cringe at myself for feeling that way. I knew I wanted to try to lessen the negative stigma attached to Alzheimer's and dementia, so I hope this book might play a small part in that. There is so much more talk about mental health these days, and our ageing population and how we care for them, and rightly so.

You are in great company, Dad, other people affected by Alzheimer's and other strains of dementia over the past decade include Glen Campbell, Robin Williams and Malcolm Young. They are also starting to make links between high-impact sports and dementia; it's a huge thing that affects so many.

If ten people read this (aside from my agent and editor) and think differently about the disease, then I would consider this book a success. If people are able to deal with the illness with a more open mind and a more open heart, I will take comfort in that. Small steps and all that!

Anyway, Dad, I always remember your love of words, of books, of talking, reading, writing. I got that from you. I remember your advice in many situations was to 'just get stuff down on paper'. I have a slick laptop but the effect is much the same. To be fair, that philosophy of yours really does have a lot to answer for. If I hadn't had some sort of outlet for my feelings ten years ago I don't know if I would have got through it. This diary might just have saved my life.

The years after you left weren't pretty; I am not unscarred, but I am here. I live and I breathe and

I love and I laugh – just as you both would have. I don't believe in the saying, 'Time is a great healer'. It's just not true. You don't 'get over' it and you don't 'move on'. The best we can hope for is that we find something to cling on to – some light, some hope, some way of dealing with loss. You don't ever get anything to fill that hole, that gaping void; you just put up some warning signs and you work around it, acknowledging that it is there but knowing that you can exist with it.

One of your other dreams, Dad, apart from your engineering prowess, was to write. I hope that this is one of those things we can do together, father and daughter, me and My Mad Dad.

Your girl, Robs x

# With thanks

Firstly, thank you, reader, for picking up this book. Your support is much appreciated not just by me but by everyone who might be affected by the issues raised in these pages. We might not have all the answers, solutions or cures, but even just a little understanding goes a long, long way.

Music has always played a big part in my life, both through good times and bad, like most people, I guess. I would like to acknowledge a few bands whose music provided the soundtrack to this period of my life. With your words and music you have made me smile and frown, laugh and cry, sing and shout, and, above all else, made me feel. And that's the point of an art form, isn't it – to make people feel something, no matter what that something is?

Initially, as a child of the 80s, I declared myself a product of American 'hair metal' or 'poodle rock', if you like, and I thrived on wailing guitars, men in Spandex and howling lyrics. School reshaped me slightly and my teenage years saw me under the Britpop spell of the 90s, shoegazing and humming along with the great unwashed. Obviously, being in Camden in the noughties, I was face to face and shoulder to shoulder with The Libertines and their counterparts, and it was thrilling to really be part of that scene as it unfolded and then unravelled.

These days I don't feel that there is a particular music 'scene' for the haters of manufactured pop, which is a shame. I am wiser for my musical education and still listen out eagerly for the next big thing, knowing that I might be too old to fully embrace it but that 'I was there' for many pivotal gigs, festivals and happenings that preceded it.

And so, in no particular order, I would like to extend thanks to the following people/bands/acts for their tremendous contribution, not just to my ears but to the ears of many.

Radiohead
Aerosmith
Whitesnake
Super Furry Animals
John Barry
Alice Cooper
Biffy Clyro
Simon and Garfunkel
U2
Smashing Pumpkins
Queens of the Stone Age
Neil Young
Talking Heads

Johnny Cash
Foo Fighters
Blur
Arcade Fire
The Libertines
Echo and The Bunnymen
Miles Davis
Bruce Springsteen
Madonna
Depeche Mode
Maximo Park
The Smiths
Pink Floyd
Slayer
Elton John
Guns N' Roses
Yeah Yeah Yeahs
Tori Amos
Kate Bush
Pantera
Feeder
Oasis
Mansun
Kiss
Counting Crows
Motörhead
Louis Armstrong and Ella Fitzgerald
Simply Red (no, not really)

There are many people who helped make this rambling

stream of consciousness into what we now know as a book. This starts with my friends who encouraged me to put my words 'out there', as it were. To my wonderful and supportive husband who only winced mildly when I announced that I would quit work to become a writer: you have no idea how amazing you are.

Then there are my Welsh wonders: my agent Cathryn who, like some intervening angel of fate, called me on Dad's birthday to offer representation; and Anna, my publisher who totally got the nuances of the story and helped polish and develop my work. You both made this happen so cheers to you and the whole team at Curtis Brown and Trapeze.

Obviously, the main theme of this book is family; they come in all shapes and sizes, and you can't choose them and you can't change them. 'Family' means different things to different people; it ebbs and flows with the years but what remains constant is the love we receive and the love that we give in return. Dad, Mum, the almighty big G, aunties, uncles, cousins and those friends so close they might as well share my blood, your love means more than you know. To the family I have, I had and am yet to receive I am truly, truly grateful.

But mainly this if for you, Dad. When I finally got my first job in London after I left university you sent me a box of Dairy Milk in the mail with a little Post-it note attached that read, 'Never let the bastards grind you down'.

And I didn't, Daddy, I didn't. x